Public Health in Postcolonial Africa

This fascinating, multi-disciplinary collection examines how public health interventions in postcolonial Africa mirror wider manifestations of power in the region.

Beyond the role of public health intervention in tackling disease and prolonging life, the book measures the social and political determinants of health which continue to exist in the postcolonial era. The volume features contributions from scholars across both the social sciences and humanities, exploring ongoing debates across a broad range of themes, including:

- Infopolitics, biopolitics and healthcare.
- Emerging infectious diseases, environment and food cultures.
- Health interventions and economic security.
- Church administration and healthcare.
- Livelihood, sex, sexuality and HIV/AIDS.

Offering a fresh and insightful understanding of health issues in this important global region, and including chapters on issues around the Covid-19 pandemic, the book will interest students and researchers across a range of disciplines, including global health, politics and African studies.

Olukayode A. Faleye is Associate Professor in History and International Studies, Edo State University, Uzairue, Edo State, Nigeria.

Tanimola M. Akande is Professor of Public Health, College of Health Sciences, University of Ilorin, Nigeria.

Inocent Moyo is Associate Professor in Geography and Environmental Studies, University of Zululand, South Africa.

Public Health in Postcolonial Africa

The Social and Political Determinants of Health

Edited by Olukayode A. Faleye,
Tanimola M. Akande and
Inocent Moyo

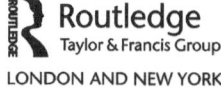

Routledge
Taylor & Francis Group

LONDON AND NEW YORK

First published 2024
by Routledge
4 Park Square, Milton Park, Abingdon, Oxon OX14 4RN

and by Routledge
605 Third Avenue, New York, NY 10158

Routledge is an imprint of the Taylor & Francis Group, an informa business

© 2024 selection and editorial matter, **Olukayode A. Faleye, Tanimola M. Akande and Inocent Moyo**; individual chapters, the contributors

The right of **Olukayode A. Faleye, Tanimola M. Akande and Inocent Moyo** to be identified as the authors of the editorial material, and of the authors for their individual chapters, has been asserted in accordance with sections 77 and 78 of the Copyright, Designs and Patents Act 1988.

British Library Cataloguing-in-Publication Data
A catalogue record for this book is available from the British Library

ISBN: 978-1-032-55128-9 (hbk)
ISBN: 978-1-032-55127-2 (pbk)
ISBN: 978-1-003-42913-5 (ebk)

DOI: 10.4324/9781003429135

Typeset in Sabon
by Apex CoVantage, LLC

Contents

Contributors

Ewomazino D. Akpor is Lecturer in Mass Communication at Edo State University, Uzairue, Edo State, Nigeria.

Peter O. Alokan is Associate Professor in Religious Studies at Joseph Ayo Babalola University, Nigeria.

Opeyemi Aluko is Lecturer in Political Science at Ajayi Crowther University, Nigeria.

Njouonap Gbetnkom Assiatou is Doctoral Researcher in Applied Foreign Languages and Commonwealth Studies at the University of Dschang, Cameroon.

Andrew Ate is Professor in Mass Communication at Edo State University, Uzairue, Edo State, Nigeria.

Solomon Awuzie is Associate Professor in African Literature at Edo State University, Uzairue, Nigeria.

Josephine Balogun is Lecturer in French, History and International Studies at Edo State University, Uzairue, Edo State, Nigeria.

Jonathan Dangana is Lecturer in Public Health at Babcock University, Nigeria.

Harriet O. Efanodor-Obeten is Associate Professor in Political Science at Edo State University, Uzairue, Edo State, Nigeria.

Basure S. Hardlife is Postdoctoral Research Fellow in Sociology and Social Anthropology at Great Zimbabwe University, Zimbabwe.

Ozekhome G. Igechi is Lecturer in Political Science at Edo State University, Uzairue, Edo State, Nigeria.

Marième Ciss is Lecturer in Sociology at Sup Management University, Senegal.

Ngetcham is Research-Lecturer in Comparative Literature at the University of Dschang Cameroon.

Arthur C. Okafor is Ernst Mach Postdoctoral Researcher at the Austrian Agency for Health and Food Safety, Vienna, Austria.

Emmanuel Okla is Lecturer in History and International Studies at Edo State University, Uzairue, Edo State, Nigeria.

Anthonia I. Otsupius is Senior Lecturer in Business Administration at Edo State University, Uzairue, Edo State, Nigeria.

Durojaiye Owoeye is Senior Lecturer in English Language at University of Lagos, Nigeria.

Acknowledgements

The initiative to publish this edited volume was conceived at the 2022 Global Health Security Conference, which was held in Singapore. The event was organized by the Global Health Security Network (GHSN) under the leadership of Professor Adam Kamradt-Scott. The Editors would like to thank the GHSN for facilitating the attendance of African scholars at the conference and for its vision for global health built on social justice.

Introduction

Public Health in Postcolonial Africa

Olukayode A. Faleye, Tanimola M. Akande, and Inocent Moyo

Public health is the governance of both natural and human endowments of society. This includes the governing of human populations, the physical environment, and even pathogens that evolve from this nature-culture nexus (Binns and Low, 2015). At the centre of public health is the need to "improve the health of the whole community with an emphasis on protection, prevention of disease, and promotion of well-being. The key themes in the concept are populations, prevention, and equity" (Binns and Low, 2015: 5). From the foregoing, it is obvious that the health security of the human population is at the centre of the public health system which elucidates the vitality of the social factor in this regard (Faleye, 2023). This is particularly the case in Africa due to its subservient position in global politics since the age of the British Empire. Indeed, the wide expanse of the landscape and cultures in Sub-Saharan Africa from Senegal to Zimbabwe were colonized spaces with serious implications for public health theory and practices. Public health means different things at different periods of world history. For instance, in the colonial era, it was an imperial tool of dominance where the disparities and inequalities in society assumed the various dichotomies of the dirt-poor disease's reservoirs symbolized by the native identity and constructed sanitary spaces of orderliness in the colonial state of disorder. These cultural forms were engendered by the science of hygiene and sanitation and its reflections on cultural identity rather than the imperial structure of power and social inequality.

In Africa, this sustained the biopolitics that saw the subjugation of the native people with little access to biomedical services and a sustainable built environment in the colonial era (Faleye and Akande, 2019). In this direction, scholars have long identified the instrumentalization of these imperial relations in biopower, and necropolitics in colonial and postcolonial environments (Fanon, 1964; Foucault, 1982; Mbembe, 2003, 2019). As these works show, public health is a product of its political geography. Hence, the political landscape is vital in understanding the preferences in the policy framework in the face of an emergency public health event. Against this backdrop, this book examines public health in postcolonial Africa from a social context. It reflects on the various contributions of the humanities and social sciences

DOI: 10.4324/9781003429135-1

to the understanding of social and political determinants of health. The contributions in this book reflect the social impact of public health interventions in Sub-Saharan Africa. Public health mirrors the manifestation of power in society. It is within this architecture that the negotiation of power between the classes in society becomes obvious. Hence, far from purely a clinical and scientific endeavour, history taught us that public health is the art of controlling both human and material resources to safeguard community health in line with the preferences of the political authorities. Thus, the composition and identity of these political authorities colour the public health architecture from a time perspective. As observed by the World Health Organization (WHO), the nature of this endeavour is characterized by the need to prevent disease and sustain life through healthy livelihoods conditioned by evidence-based ideas about the organization of society across strata of governance which include public, private, and individual levels.

In the context of the colonial historiography and politics of public health, the early 21st century marked a significant upsurge in the output of African humanists and social scientists. While this is remarkable, most of the existing studies are buried in the dust without forging a strong link to the advancement of medical theory and public health practices in postcolonial Africa. Hence, the title of this volume centring on the chronological framework of the "postcolonial" is not a mistake but an articulation of changing power dynamics in Sub-Saharan Africa as it manifests through the often-invisible hands of public health. This is a multi-disciplinary endeavour linking the past to the present. Moreover, the volume complements the scientific underpinnings of public health policies and practices by unveiling the various social dimensions and dynamics of health interventions. While the volume's thematic content is not fulsome in capturing all the episodes of health emergencies and interventions in postcolonial Africa, it provides a reference point on the social morphology of health and wellness as well as sickness and illness based on major public health episodes in contemporary African societies after colonial rule. Beyond the role of public health intervention in apprehending disease outbreaks and prolonging life through access to the required infrastructure, this volume measures the social cost effect of the public health regulations and the lessons thereof.

The term "postcolonial" as used in this book is at once periodical, transitional, and methodological. It is periodical and transitional because it marks a departure from the colonial era and a transition to the postcolonial era where Africans took over the mantle of political governance of their country. Here, how the major change from a Eurocentric imperial structure to Afrocentric governance impacts public health infrastructure in Africa is worthy of scholarly inquiry. This poses a methodological change in the context of the generation of new sources of public health data in a new environment after the Age of Empire. Nevertheless, in a globalizing world, putting local public health scenario into the global context unveils the histories and geopolitics of health beyond the national boundaries. This book shows how these dynamics reflect local and global changes in the form of public health governance, diplomacy, and the access to health infrastructure. Furthermore, the term "postcolonial" is intended to illuminate the intention of this book in interrogating the existing dominant knowledge on public health and the inclusion (or lack of it) of marginalized indigenous knowledge about health and well-being. This is important given the present coloniality of knowledge. The institutionalization of this imperial knowledge system that seeks to create an uneven space in which the dominant power in societies confiscates the right to live undermines the ideals of the humanity. Scholars have examined the biopolitical view of human existence where targeted individuals' bodies are legally commoditized and disposed of based on identity framing (Fanon, 1964; Foucault, 1982). Otherwise, a necropolitics that rationalizes the legal right to genocidal pruning of a target population through draconian regulations camouflaged as health policies is untenable in an increasingly globalized world (Mbembe, 2003, 2019).

The contributions to this volume are disciplinarily diverse straddling the arts to the social sciences with reflections on the pure sciences. In Chapter 1, Harriet O. Efanodor-Obeten and Ozekhome G. Igechi address the politics of healthcare reforms in postcolonial Nigeria. The study traces the foundation of the postcolonial healthcare system to the Walter-Harkness Ten Year Plan between 1946 and 1955, which instituted the metropolitan forms of healthcare services at the eve of Nigerian independence. This was an integrative scheme built on the urban planning formular of the late 1920s, thereby incorporating the ideas of environmental sanitation, hygiene, water supply, and provision of hospitals and dispensaries at both urban and rural areas in Nigeria. The authors argue that the healthcare reforms in postcolonial Nigeria became integrated into the national development plans at independence with the aim to address the inequitable healthcare system earlier instituted by the colonial administration. As Harriet O. Efanodor-Obeten and Ozekhome G. Igechi show, the Nigerian political structure and method of public administration dictated the performance of public health reforms and policies in the postcolonial era.

Chapter 2 discusses the climate change-public health nexus from multiple dimensions including socio-ecological conflicts, extractive systems, social inequality, cross-border migration, and political violence in Sub-Saharan Africa. It showcases the dynamics of climate change from the lenses of power asymmetry, uneven allocation of resources, and sustainable development in the region. Drawing useful insight from postcolonial theories of biopolitics and necropolitics, the chapter uncovers the complexities of climate change in the context of the political economy of adaptive systems in Sub-Saharan Africa. Here, Olukayode A. Faleye, Tanimola M. Akande, and Inocent Moyo argue that environmental resource challenges, adaptative violence, are accentuated by the power structures in society with serious implications for public health in postcolonial Africa. In Chapter 3, Marième Ciss discussed the public health policies and implementation in postcolonial Senegal in the context of equity in access to healthcare services. Marieme argues that vain political rhetoric on public health intervention masks the failure of the state to fulfil its function of social protection of the populace. The analysis is hinged on the role of health committees, social hospital services, and free healthcare policies, including the Sesame Plan and the UHC. The study unveils the necropolitics of health interventions that designate the grave as abode of the poorest people in postcolonial Senegal.

Chapter 4 shows that the politics of spatial demography impact rural-urban inequalities and health interventions in Sub-Saharan Africa. While the extant literature emphasizes the importance of demographic data in health interventions, this chapter advances a socio-political determinant of health infrastructure in Sub-Saharan Africa. Particular attention is directed to the management of Lassa fever and Ebola Virus Disease outbreaks in Sub-Saharan African with a focus on postcolonial Lagos. In Chapter 5, Peter O. Alokan and Opeyemi Aluko examined the socio-economic impact of Covid-19 pandemic on the church and Nigerian Christians with a particular reference to the Christ Apostolic Church. While the chapter unveils the impact of public health measures on the church administration with regard to financial difficulties and the stifling spiritualism, it also reflects the place of the church as an agency of public health in local communities. In this vein, Alokan and Aluko unveil the relationship between the Nigerian state, church, and society in a time of the pandemic. In Chapter 6, Josephine Balogun and Emmanuel Okla analyse the intervention of the Catholic Church in the area of healthcare in Nigeria. Indeed, Chapter 6 focuses on the role of the church in abating the scourge of HIV/AIDS, Ebola Virus Disease, and Covid-19 pandemic in Nigeria. This form of social evangelization is often forgotten in the public health literature, whereas it unveils the importance of the church in health intervention.

In Chapter 7, Basure S. Hardlife analyses the nexus between sex, sexuality, and Asian aphrodisiacs in Zimbabwe. In dismantling discriminatory and anti-African attitudes of the colonial system, the chapter shows that the distribution and consumption of aphrodisiac is a reflection of the postcolonial valuation of sex and sexuality which constitute a public health challenge, if the cosmopolitan nature of the distribution and consumption networks of these products is brought to the fore. Chapter 8 examines the nexus between HIV/AIDS and the media in Nigeria. According to Andrew Ate, Ewomazino D. Akpor, and Anthonia I. Otsupius, the mass media promotes promiscuities that facilitate the spread of the virus. On the other hand, it aids publicity, advocacy, and information dissemination aimed at preventing and reducing the spread of HIV/AIDS Nigeria. Andrew Ate, Ewomazino D. Akpor, and Anthonia I. Otsupius posit that finding a middle ground amidst this complexity is vital to the control of deadly viruses. This reveals the mass media as an important social determinant of sexuality and sexually transmitted diseases in postcolonial Nigeria.

Language and literature are mediums of public opinion. It is against this background that Ngetcham and Njouonap Gbetnkom Assiatou, in Chapter 9, examine how local medicine practitioners contribute to healing diseases in postcolonial Cameroon. This chapter underpinned by African literary texts shows the writing back of the coloniality of medical practices in postcolonial Africa through the endurance of African traditional medicine in healing the Africa's ill. It argues that beyond the obliteration of colonial presence in postcolonial medical realities in Africa, medical postcolonialism combines the benevolent aspects of orthodox and traditional medicines in forging sustainable holistic medical practices in postcolonial Africa.

In Chapter 10, Solomon Awuzie explores the evidence of mental disorders by diagnosing Nigerian literary writers through the structure of their written text. It shows that the postcolonial Nigerian poetry has already revealed the poets' maddened discontentment with his immediate realities, but this study provides evidence as well as reasons for this and engages the personas' chaotic existential situations, which are occasioned by ethnic hatred and poor governance. With the analysis of selected postcolonial Nigerian poetry, the imbalance in Nigerian social existence is stressed, and it is discovered that there is the proliferation of the symptoms of paranoia in postcolonial Nigerian poetry as compared to the symptoms of schizophrenia as a result of this. The chapter argues that the reflection on the personas as paranoiac stresses the effect of necropolitics in the Nigerian socio-space and harps on the need to engage with the evils of ethnic hatred and poor governance that are responsible for these symptoms of mental stress and emotional frustration. In Chapter 11, Durojaiye Owoeye discusses the idea of Trumpism and the necropolitics of the Covid-19 pandemic with reflection on the implications and relevance of the American experience to Sub-Saharan Africa. It shows President Trump's idiosyncratic temperaments and hypersensitivity to a political ideology in the face of Covid-19 and how this influences health interventions in the United States. Finally, the conclusion considers the global implications of the volume for postcolonial approaches to health, beyond Africa.

References

Binns, C. and Low, W.-Y. (2015). What Is Public Health? *Asia Pacific Journal of Public Health*, 27(1): 5–6.

Faleye, O.A. (2023). COVID-19 Pandemic, Geopolitics of Health and Security Entanglement in West Africa. In Moyo, I. and Ndlovu-Gatsheri, S.J. (Eds.) *COVID-19 Pandemic and the Politics of Life*. London: Routledge.

Faleye, O.A. and Akande, T.M. (2019). Beyond "White Medicine": Bubonic Plague and Health Interventions in Colonial Lagos. *Gesnerus: Swiss Journal of the History of Medicine and Sciences*, 76(1): 90–110.

Fanon, F. (1964). *Toward the African Revolution*. New York: Grove Press.

Foucault, M. (1982). The Subject and Power. *Critical Inquiry*, 8(4): 777–795.

Mbembe, J.A. (2003). Necropolitics. *Public Culture*, 15(1): 11–40.

Mbembe, J.A. (2019). *Necropolitics*. Durham: Duke University Press.

Part I

Healthcare Policy, Politics of Space and Social Justice

1 Politics of Healthcare Reform in Postcolonial Nigeria

Harriet O. Efanodor-Obeten and Ozekhome G. Igechi

Introduction

One of the major developmental indicators of every nation is the rate at which citizens access healthcare services. This is true because the socio-economic and political development of a people will be practically impossible without the government making the needed resources available to protect the health of its population. It has been argued, by Fogel (1991), that the Industrial Revolution in England was successful, at least in part, because they were able to curtail morbidity and mortality, which at the time were high. The defeat of several contagious diseases coupled with an improvement in the nutrition level of the whole population in Britain meant that the nation could face the challenge of development. A healthy population is more likely to increase productivity, strengthen people's capability and their propensity for savings and investments as well as promote other behaviours and tendencies that encourage productivity. On the other hand, a strong economic framework encourages the development of a sound healthcare system.

A very strong economy can easily aggregate resources to finance environmental and other sanitary components of the healthcare system and is also more able to engage in sensitization concerning immunization, screening and vaccination. For example, in the context of the Covid-19 pandemic, countries must aggregate the needed funds to procure vaccines for their populations. Again, social development in education requires a concomitant effort to improve the health conditions of the population to improve not just nutrition but also reproductive health. However, as will be seen later, not all macroeconomic growth ambitions positively impact on healthcare. This is especially true for developing economies, and as will be seen in Nigeria, in the context of structural adjustment where policies had negative ramifications for healthcare services (Muiu, 2002). Indeed, the post-independence history of Africa's most populous nation is one of failed aspirations with the health system not doing any better than other sectors.

The poor performance of the healthcare system in Nigeria has often led to continuous reformation, with political leadership and their bureaucratic counterparts trying to make the healthcare system function properly.

DOI: 10.4324/9781003429135-3

Following independence, the realization by the political class that there is a correlation between a sound health system and economic development led them to engage in a number of reforms in the health sector. While these efforts are commendable, they nevertheless have been unable to bring about the needed transformation that the nation's health system deserves. This is because successive governments, military and civilian, in the post-independence history of Nigeria have politicized public policies to the detriment of efficiency and public interest. That is why the nation performs poorly in most critical healthcare indices. For example, average life expectancy at birth is 55.12 years, while under-five mortality rate stands at 117.2 per 1000 live births (UNICEF, 2021). This seems an indictment on the sincerity of the political class in the reform process within the healthcare system.

The politicization of health policies has meant that there has been poor allocation of resources and the governments at all levels are culpable (Faleye, 2023). Provision of healthcare to the underclass is one of the most effective ways of pursuing social protection and inclusive growth. When the poor can access healthcare, they not only become economically empowered but also begin to feel a sense of socio-political belonging that aids national integration. Some of the healthcare reforms that have been historically deployed in Nigeria to act as social protection mechanisms include National Health Insurance Scheme (NHIS), Basic Health Services Scheme (BHSS), National Immunization Coverage Scheme (NICS), Midwives Service Scheme (MSS), Primary Healthcare Under One Roof (PHCUOR), Revitalization of Primary Health Care and the Nigerian Pay for Performance Scheme (P4P). It is in the light of the above background that this chapter scrutinizes the politics of healthcare reforms in postcolonial Nigeria. This discourse is driven, at least in part, by Michel Foucault's conception of biopolitics especially as rendered by Campbell and Sitze (2013). The biopolitical has become a very critical philosophical pedestal as states continue to seek avenues to advance the health and well-being of their populations. At the outset we engage some conceptual themes for a deeper and better understanding of the issues. We then explore healthcare reforms in Nigeria through different epochs. The chapter exits with a template that can improve healthcare services in Nigeria.

Conceptual Discourse

Politics as a concept is highly 'loaded' because it does not have a universally accepted definition. This is partly because different authors and writers see the state and society in different lights and interpret governance decisions differently. For example, some writers see the state and society as overlapping, while others have a rigid and clear-cut differentiation of the two. Indeed, among scholars there is hardly unanimity on what the concept of politics means. However, there have been various attempts at defining politics. Nwabuzor and Mueller (1985) observe that politics dominate all levels of society, whether horizontal or vertical. This holistic approach reflects the thinking of those who equate the society with state. Thus, politics permeates the society at large, as the struggle to preside over resources and status can occur in the market and the church. Leftwich (2008: 6) aligns with this position when he argued that 'politics is best conceptualized as consisting of all the many activities of cooperation, conflict and negotiation involved in decisions about the use, production and distribution of resources'. This position sees everything within society, development inclusive, as being inherently political.

On the other hand, a number of theorists have embraced the notion that politics only has to do with situations in which an agent has the authority to dispense resources, status, power, resources and other values. According to Easton (1965) politics involves the authoritative allocation of values. Gabriel (2017) emphasizes the Eastonian tradition when he argued that decisions are best enforced when they are binding for an entire people living within a territory. When the community is in unison about the values and the justice and enforcement system, it is easy for it to then apply rules. This position is in tandem with the belief that the sphere of the state is different from that of the larger society. The state is that formal organization that is responsible for applying rules as spelt out in the constitution. Thus, politics drives public policies in the formal arena of government. The Eastonian conceptualization of politics remains very influential within the discipline.

Public healthcare has been defined as that part of public policy that involves the administration of what people eat, drink and how society live together without diseases (Porta, 2014). Public healthcare is inextricably linked with the environmental, social, political, economic, educational, occupational and medical aspects of the society. This is not quite elusive to grasp as, for example, the environment in which we live may generate sanitary problems with huge repercussions for the health and well-being of the citizens. Social relations in the physical space that we share can be a source of diseases. In the context of the Covid-19 pandemic it has become advisable for people to keep social distance in order to reduce the rate at which the virus spread (Burrows and Engelke, 2020). Politics brings the needed coordination that public policy requires to make the health sector good for the people. The economy is a critical component public health. The same goes for education, occupation and the medical arena, which is central to the health and well-being of the people. Winslow (1920: 4) provides a classic definition of public healthcare, referring to it as the

> science and art of preventing diseases, prolonging life and promoting health and efficiency through organized community effort for the sanitation of the environment; the control of communicable infections; the education of the individual in personal hygiene; the organization of medical and nursing services for the early diagnosis and preventive treatment of diseases; and the development of social machinery to give everyone a standard of living adequate for the maintenance of health and organizing these benefits as to enable every citizen to realize his birth right of health and longevity.

This comprehensive conceptualization of healthcare summarizes the core themes that governments everywhere engage with as they try to ensure that their citizens' well-being is not compromised. The public healthcare system has also been defined as an organizational framework for the distribution or servicing of the healthcare needs of a community (Asuzu, 2004). This system is a complex admixture of different inter-related components cutting across medical, environmental, economic, political and social spheres.

It is popular to put down the necessity of reforms to rational political or ideological discoveries that challenge the existing orthodoxy. This will then lead to practical policy changes relevant to improving the conditions of the particular field. Politics as an endeavour must necessarily be treated as an intellectual concern which must deploy straightforward rationalism in public policy decision making, implementation and evaluation. Different factors may be responsible for government to engage in reform. Some include the changing role of the state, technological development and changing nature of globalization (Ball, 1998). In the context of public healthcare, reforms often mean the formulation, implementation and evaluation of a specific public policy concerning health which involves to some degree the role of the state and some contribution from the private sector as represented by market forces. At any point in time a government can consider tweaking the degree of intervention it engages with a specific public service. The healthcare sector is one such arena where a decision can be made to carry out comprehensive or incremental changes with a view to increasing productivity and efficiency.

In the political process, reform is carried out when there is a tendency to believe that present policy practices are not meeting the needs and aspirations of society. Under such circumstances, a cost-benefit analysis or a linear means-ends construct is deployed rationally to improve what the government is doing. When it appears to policy makers that current standards fall below expectations, they are likely to change them for better ones with the expectation that the situation will improve. However, beyond this rational desire to uplift governance performance, reform may come because the hegemonic segment of the ruling class desires a change. Personal, partisan and other primordial reasons may lead political leadership to engage in reforms (Edelman, 1988). While this is clearly a deviation from good governance norms and practice, the tendency is nevertheless sometimes common in Sub-Saharan African policy circles where there may be some public officials with the intent to pervert the public policy process. Reforms within Nigeria's healthcare system have had several reforms since independence. It is to these issues this chapter now turns.

Healthcare Reforms in the Context of Development Planning

In the period immediately following independence, healthcare reforms in Nigeria were inculcated into National Development Plans framework. The idea was to ensure that political power birthed a strong and healthy population and a situation that will strengthen state power for effective development (Sinnerbrink, 2005). Prior to that time, modern medicine was alien to the indigenous people of what later became known as Nigeria (Anaemene and Aworawo, 2014). However, with first colonialism and then outright independence, Nigeria gradually embraced Western medicine as it is known today. It has been noted that the health sector suffered significant neglect at the onset of colonial rule in Nigeria as the majority of the population depended on traditional medicine even in the colonial capital – Lagos (Faleye, 2019). Subsequently, historians have shown that the earliest elements of health reform were characterized by interventions in infectious disease outbreaks and urban planning following disease outbreaks such as the plague in colonial Lagos (Olukoju, 2003; Faleye, 2017). Thus, the first concrete attempt at health sector reform was the Walter-Harkness Ten-Year Plan of 1946–1955 launched by the British colonial administration (Anaemene and Aworawo, 2014). With this plan, health services in Nigeria were never the same again. It perhaps completely revolutionized the sector as metropolitan methods of healthcare gradually started to become popular and they existed side by side with trado-medical healthcare methods. During this time, the colonial government proposed a plan in which there will be progressive development of healthcare infrastructures. In this respect there was a steady improvement in environmental hygiene, childcare, availability of portable water, the expansion of hospital and dispensary services and the up-scaling of preventive medicine at the rural level.

It was during the period immediately before independence that the University College Hospital (UCH), Ibadan, was established, and it became the first quality tertiary health manpower training institution in the country. Subsequently, the government established more health facilities mainly in towns like Lagos, Enugu, Markudi, Sokoto and Jos. At independence, these were the health infrastructures that the home government had to rely on. Thus, beginning from 1960, healthcare reforms started to be inculcated into successive National Development plans or better still as part of specific health issues. The first National Development Plan, which was to run from 1962 until 1968, had the objective of promoting industrial development, the establishment of modern medical centres in the major cities and the building of dispensaries and maternities in a few rural areas (FGN, 1970). This objective was noble as political leadership discovered that there can be no meaningful development if the health and well-being of citizens are not well protected.

The healthcare deliverables in the Second National Development Plan (1970–1974) were crafted, in part, to ameliorate some of the deficiencies in the first National Development Plan. The overarching national objectives formulated in the second National Development Plan include the establishment of: a free and democratic society; a just and egalitarian society; a united, strong and self-reliant nation; a great and dynamic economy; and a bright land full of opportunities (FGN, 1970). Within the context of a free, just and egalitarian society, the healthcare sector was expected to promote the wellness of citizens. In this direction, there was a conscious attempt at drawing out a comprehensive national healthcare policy that will address 'basic health service scheme, disease control, efficient utilization of health resources, medical research and health planning and management' (Anaemene, 2016: 6). In terms of expansion of existing health infrastructure across the country, reforms carried out during the period were fairly successful.

At the federal level, the required resources were made available for the University Teaching Hospitals in Lagos, Ibadan and Enugu and for the Specialist Hospitals in Benin, Enugu and Ilorin, which were duly expanded. The Bed space and carrying capacity of the University College Ibadan was increased to 520, and the Lagos University Teaching Hospital was expanded, with its Dentistry Unit upgraded. Also the OPD Ward Theatre, the Radio diagnosis and physical medicine units were completed. In line with the competitive federalist spirit of the time, the states made giant strides in the healthcare reforms as many keyed into the development at the national level. At the state level, over 300 healthcare and maternity centres were established as the nation was making use of a financial whirlwind occasioned by increase in oil revenue following the Yom Kippur war in the Middle East. Yet these achievements were to some extent limited. There were still shortages of manpower and critical health personnel while there was also no clear-cut delineation as regarding the levels of government. Healthcare infrastructures were still absent in many rural areas, places in the outer reaches that appeared to be beyond the reach of public policy.

The Third National Development Plan (1975–1980) had the overriding objective of directing reform in the healthcare sector towards Basic Health Services Schemes. The primary goal was to increase the number of people who had access to modern healthcare from a meagre 25% to 60%. The Basic Health Service Scheme as enshrined in the Third Development Plan aimed to achieve the following: to embark on the provision of adequate and efficient healthcare facilities for Nigerians; to correct the imbalance in the spatial distribution of health infrastructure directed at preventive and curative measures; to provide infrastructure for all preventive healthcare services like communicable diseases, family health, nutrition and similar matters; to put in place an healthcare system that is best suited to local conditions in view of the available technology (FGN, 1975). The healthcare reform that came with the Third National Development Plan was comprehensive, and there was an allocation of 20 million naira to the fight against malaria. There were also different collaborations with International Organizations and NGOs for vaccination, for example against smallpox. The period saw the increase in the number of federally managed Teaching Hospitals, where health personnel were trained. However, there was still no clear-cut policy framework for healthcare which continued to be lumped together with sundry issues. Again, professional manpower was still minimal and there was lack of policy to effectively share responsibilities among the levels of government.

The healthcare reforms that came with the Fourth National Development Plan (1981–1985) continued to place some premium on the Basic Health Service Scheme, which ironically had been receiving little attention from the government. This was so because even with the Fourth Development Plan the federal government continued to concentrate on the development of Teaching and Specialist Hospitals across the nation. This was clearly evidenced in the budgetary allocation as captured in the nation's financial documents. For example, while a total of N862.40 million was spent on infrastructural and personnel development in the Teaching and Specialist Hospitals, only N101.00 million was voted for the Basic Health Service Scheme and other similar programmes during the period (Anaemene, 2016). The priority of government was therefore easy to see, however curious the whole agenda was. There is not much to be said about the reforms that accompanied the Fifth National Development Plan (1987–1991) as the period dovetailed with the adoption of the primary healthcare strategy and the National Health Policy in 1988. In any case, the nation had already embraced the Structural Adjustment Programme (SAP) as there appeared a strong desire by political leaders to seek external borrowing with serious ramification for every sector of the economy.

Healthcare Reforms During Structural Adjustment Programme (SAP)

The postcolonial history concerning any aspect of the Nigerian state can hardly be discussed without reference to the economic crises of the 1980s and the adoption of the Structural Adjustment Programme (SAP) with serious ramifications for socio-economic activities. Several commentators have put down the 'inevitability' of economic structural adjustments to the disarticulation of the economy, a mono-cultural economy and the global economic crises of the 1980s (Osaghae, 2002). In the face of these negative tendencies, coupled with elitist prebendalism, the nation was close to its knees in the middle of the 1980s as public finance suffered serious crises. The President Shagari administration (1979–1983) had mooted the idea of SAP and indeed took two loans from the World Bank and the International Monetary Fund (IMF). The adoption of SAP was, in part, due to pressures from creditors. Briefly, some of the basic elements of SAP as described by Synge (1993: 44–45) included: fiscal deficit reduction, stimulation of domestic production, devaluation of the local currency (naira), rationalization of customs tariff, deregulation of the banking system, removal of subsidies on petroleum products, water, electricity and so on, and the privatization and commercialization of public enterprises. Indeed, liberalization of this nature followed Michel Foucault's argument that 'power is everywhere' such that the people become the ultimate domain for which power ought to rightly be exercised.

These activities in the realm of the economy had serious consequences for public spending and indeed for healthcare financing. The SAP practically meant a reduction in the degree of state intervention in the process of resource spending and control within the society. And to sustain the project, countries have to meet certain conditionalities tied to the aforementioned elements of SAP. Otherwise, creditors will no longer play their role of providing funds and technical support. SAP was gradually introduced with the initial stage of national economic emergency beginning 1 October 1985 (Osaghae, 2002). A number of measures were deployed to increase government revenue, especially from different types of taxes and levies. This was in addition to the fact that the government had reduced its sphere of public spending, as it pushed for privatization and commercialization of some public concerns. All of these were to have serious ramifications for healthcare spending since the government was now unwilling to engage in big spending as there was the need to meet the terms of the negotiation that was made with external creditors.

The existential implementation of SAP, with its negative conditionalities, posed serious challenge to health sector spending and the healthcare of Nigerians (Popoola, 1993; Anaemene, 2016). In the period following the adoption of SAP, Nigeria, started to rely on loans and borrowings to fund many capital projects and programmes, including those domiciled in the health sector. This of course logically followed the fact that public spending had to be done in tandem with the conditions which foreign creditors had stipulated. There was now a gradual movement away from direct government intervention in healthcare provision to a situation in which government efforts were supported by the private sector. This led to the introduction of certain fees that were hitherto not charged, and there was also the resort to some other templates like public-private partnerships and the contracting out to private concerns all in the hope that public healthcare delivery will improve. This liberalization of the public space informed the reforms that were carried out in the health sector during this period.

To put this government's gradual withdrawal from public health spending during the time into proper perspective, some key indicators can be used to illustrate this. Public health spending as a proportion of government budget expenditure fell from an average of 3.5% in the 1970s to an average of 2% in the 1980s and 1990s (Anaemene, 2016). This shift in public health spending had serious implications for public hospitals generally and the resource persons operating within these institutions. The consequence was frequent crises in the health sector which manifested in dilapidated structures, shortages of drugs, frequent industrial crises and the emigration of specialist health workers who had not only become de-motivated but also disillusioned. It thus became fashionable for Nigerian medical doctors to travel out of the country in search of greener pastures. The introduction of cost-recovery devices meant that free medical services had been abolished. It was during this period that there was a huge motivation for the establishment of private healthcare services due essentially to the apparent fall in the quality of public health institutions (Ogunbekun, Ogunbekun, and Orobatan, 1999).

The advent of the Structural Adjustment Programme (SAP) in the middle of the 1990s came with the attempt at reducing government public spending. This was not peculiar to the health sector as other areas had similar challenges. The coming onboard of private health service providers as well as the increasing commercialization of healthcare services was seen as a major impediment to the quest for the enthronement of an egalitarian society. In most societies, healthcare alongside education are some of the ways through which government pursues inclusive growth. That is why healthcare is often subsidized by the government. Quality healthcare is expensive, and because wellness and longevity are key indices for gauging average life expectancy, it becomes important that states subsidize it so that their people can live a better and healthy life that will encourage productivity.

It is based on these crises that a summit was held at the close of the 20th century to critically evaluate them and to search for solutions. The National Health Summit was convened in 1995 to look for and chart a new course for healthcare services in Nigeria. At the time, Nigeria had lost credibility in the eyes of the international community. It was therefore natural that critical Bretton Woods stakeholders like the World Bank and the IMF were no longer favourable to Nigeria in negotiations concerning the Structural Adjustment Programme. This accounts for why the nation had to look inwards with a view to coming up with home-grown solutions. The Federal Ministry of Health revamped the National Health Policy in 1996, even though this revised health policy did not receive the needed endorsement at the time. What followed two years later was the attempt to return the nation to democratic and civilian dispensation with emphasis on the rule of law. This was eventually achieved in 1999, with retired General Olusegun Obasanjo becoming the president.

Healthcare Reforms in the Fourth Republic

The military regime of General Abdulsalami Abubakar handed political power to a democratically elected government on 29 May 1999. This civilian government was led by Chief Olusegun Obasanjo (Rtd), who himself had been a military Head of State between 1976 and 1979. In 2001, Primary Health Care programme came on board. It was constructed via the political wards as the units (Aregbeshola, 2021). The president had the intention of pulling the nation by the scruff of its neck towards development. Several novel Departments, Parastatal and Agencies (DPAs) came on board. The Economic and Financial Crimes Commission, for example, was one such reform in the criminal justice system. In the healthcare sector the National Health Insurance Scheme (NHIS), eventually got the legal, resources and infrastructural backing needed for operations. The government, in fulfilling its campaign promise to the people, embarked on a lot of developmental efforts to pull citizens out of poverty, squalor and lack. It was a general consensus among historians and writers on development concerning the Nigerian state that the military did not do enough to help the citizens, and as such it fell to the democratic governments of the Fourth Republic to pull the nation out of the socio-economic crises.

Sequel to the above, the Obasanjo Presidency, in 2003, embarked on a large-scale health sector reform with the initial phase running between 2004 and 2007 (FMOH, 2004). This health reform was situated within the administration's overarching National Economic and Empowerment Development Strategy (NEEDS). The major objective of this reform programme was to improve the existential living conditions of Nigerians and turn around the vicious cycle of hunger, poverty, deprivation, ill-health and every other indices of underdevelopment. The reform agenda articulated certain fundamentals for sustainable healthcare development, such as raising the level of government intervention in the sector, improving the national health system and its administration, clamping down on the problem of diseases, effective administration of available health resources, making access to healthcare open to the underclass, raising user awareness and encouraging community participation in the public healthcare terrain, and to encourage workable partnership with non-state institutions inside and outside Nigeria (FMOH, 2004).

In the context of Fourth Republic politics, governance has become one of the core issues facing healthcare reforms. A major sore point in public health governance in the nation is the absence of coordination in the response to the most critical health challenges. For example, there was apparent lack of synergy among critical stakeholders in the health sector across the three tiers of government. There is ample evidence to show that the constitution did not clearly delineate the sphere of influence of the three tiers of government, federal-state-local, in the healthcare sector (FMOH, 2004; Anaemene, 2016). There has always been a situation in which there is not a well-structured role-responsibility nexus as it concerns the contribution of these three tiers of government to the public healthcare system. The constitution does not clearly stipulate it, and for a federal state this is an anomaly as there ought to be a lucid sharing of responsibilities to reflect the powers of the centre and the component units. The role of the third tier, that is, local government, will then be clearly spelt out.

The local government, which ought to be the axle on which primary healthcare is driven, seems not to have the concomitant power to carry out that function. In much of the current Fourth Republic, the powers and indeed the resources of local governments have been usurped by the states through various ways. First, local governments are often not democratically elected. The governors have a vice grip on the various state electoral commissions as they control not just their finance but also the pleasure of appointing their senior officials. On the basis of this evidence, it becomes practically impossible for local government chairpersons to control the resources that are allocated to them. Second, the financial culture of operating a joint State-local government account does not help reforms in the third tier of government. This tendency of routing money meant for local governments through the states gives state governors the opportunity to divert some of the resources meant for the local governments.

One of the greatest breakthroughs in healthcare reforms in the Fourth Republic was the inauguration of the National Health Insurance Scheme (NHIS) in 2005. It is incisive to note that the scheme had been in the pipeline for much of the post-independence history of the nation, but its emergence was frustrated and delayed by politics. While the idea behind it was conceptualized at independence, political instability did not allow it to birth as several ad-hoc bodies were put in place – for example, National Council on Health, Community Based Health Financing Schemes and Social Health Insurance-at different points in time (Omoruan, Bamidele, and Philips, 2009). The Obasanjo administration eventually summoned the needed political will to bring it to light. The NHIS receives premium and provides healthcare services for formal sector workers (public and private). The scheme, however, has been criticized as being against the spirit of inclusive growth. Formal sector employees in Nigeria are less than 40% of the total population (Anaemene, 2016). Again, irrespective of the establishment of the scheme, about 90% of healthcare services are still provided for by user fees. In essence the better part of the population does not see the NHIS as being of real utility.

Subsequent administrations since the Obasanjo years have not carried out significant reforms.

The Yar'adua, Jonathan and Buhari dispensations have carried out health policies in the context of existing templates from the Obasanjo years. However, some of these reforms require brief highlight. In 2009, the Midwives Service Scheme (MSS) was established to tackle issues of manpower for PHC to increase access to skilled birth delivery and through this reduce maternal deaths. In 2010 the Nigeria's State Health Investment Project (NSHIP) was launched by the World Bank in synergy with the government to improve the delivery of high-impact services in some selected states in Nigeria. In 2011 the primary healthcare under one roof (PHCUOR) was birthed in order to integrate PHC services. In 2012, there was the SURE-P maternal and child-care initiative to cushion the effect of subsidy removal on the poor. Later in 2012 there was the save one million lives initiative, which operated in the PHC services. In 2017, the National Health Act (NHA) eventually came on board, as a pilot programme in three states: Abia, Osun and Niger. In 2018, Nigeria government embarked on the Basic Health Care Provision Fund (BHCPF), with a national steering committee to handle its initial operations.

Healthcare Reforms in Nigeria: Problems and Prospects

Upon careful consideration of the various healthcare reforms and policies in the postcolonial history of the nation, Africa's biggest democracy has largely struggled to meet the healthcare needs of its teeming population. While some aspects of the reforms are commendable as they have been useful, the entirety of the attempt at enthroning a decent healthcare regime has largely fallen short of expectations. The basic objective of every healthcare reform is to improve the existential living conditions of citizens, to make access to quality services in the hospitals and to effectively give people the opportunity to live in an environment where they can become their best self. Decades of neglect of the local government as a tier of the Nigerian state is one reason for the abysmal performance of many primary healthcare institutions. Added to this is the fact that their autonomy has always been in jeopardy, leaving many of their responsibilities hanging. The end game therefore is a reduction in the quality of the services emanating from primary healthcare institutions across the nation. As a result of this scenario, the various reforms in the health sector have failed to yield the requisite fruits since the fundamental governance structures necessary to complement reforms were not well articulated.

Beyond structural deficiencies concerning intergovernmental relations within Nigeria's federal system, the culture of corruption has also posed a serious problem to the quest for a better healthcare system via reforms in the sector. Corruption, prebendalism and avarice on the part of politicians and other top government functionaries have often meant that the resources needed to carry out reforms are frittered away through different modes of fleecing. This partly accounts for why the various reforms have fallen short of the expected outcomes and why the nation's health sector has remained in a state of comatose. While the corruption conundrum cannot be said to have emanated within the democratic governance milieu (it was there during military regimes), it nevertheless has become exacerbated, with the clear encroachment of the autonomy of state institutions by a political class that is hell-bent on pursuing politics as a zero-sum game. Burgeoning corruption within Nigeria's governance space has often made the nation perform poorly in Transparency International's yearly Corruption Perception Index (CPI). In the 2020 survey, of 180 countries, Nigeria ranked an abysmal 149 (TI, 2021), a reflection of existential reality in a nation where the political class hoarded COVID-19 palliatives and have often diverted resources meant for the well-being of its citizens.

The consequence of the anomaly plaguing the healthcare system in Nigeria is the inability of a large population within the nation to access public health service. The average national accessibility to health facility in Nigeria is below 55% (Anaemene, 2016) which falls well below the UNICEF (2000) recommended figure of 65% for African countries. It is worthy of note that people who reside in urban areas tend to have more access to healthcare facilities as these facilities are often located in such places. The fate of rural dwellers continues to be mired in uncertainty as there is often less governmental presence in such areas. This is due to the epileptic nature of Primary Health Care institutions in most places in the nation, and as has been established above, this can be largely traced to the relegation of the third tier of government in the context of Nigeria's federal system of government. The usurpation of both the powers and resources of local governments has meant that they have often been unable to carry out their statutory functions. This situation must change if there is to be an improvement in Primary Health Care service delivery.

This discourse will not be complete without a word or two on the National Health Insurance Authority Act (2022), which became law under the administration of President Muhammadu Buhari. The major innovation in the novel NHIA, which is to replace the erstwhile NHIS, is that it pushes for the universal application of health insurance to all sections of the Nigerian legal populace, making it mandatory for all citizens irrespective of whether they operate in the formal or informal arena. To be sure, the new Act does not render invalid any previous decisions or operations that were duly undertaken under the old order – be they privileges, rights or liabilities (Fatunmole, 2022). This is perhaps to ensure continuity in the governance of the health sector and to engender stability in socio-economic development. As such, in line with the precepts of the NHIS, the law provides that all poor people be provided with health insurance.

The NHIA Act is supported by a standing council which guides and regulates its operations, and there is also a provision for Third Party Administrators (TPAs) that can spread the health insurance net and allow more people to enjoy the benefit of the Act. These provisions are perhaps to avoid the drawbacks that were inherent in the NHIS scheme, whose coverage was very low and excluded many poor non-public sector employees, as it was suggested that less than 10% of the over 217 million Nigerians were covered in the scheme. Furthermore it was always the case for the health sector to experience brain drain as a number of medical personnel often left for greener pastures elsewhere due essentially to the miserly budget allocation to the health sector which often leave Nigerian hospitals in decrepit conditions alongside the poor remuneration of health sector workers whether of the Nigerian Medical Doctors variant or the Joint Health Sector Union (JOHESU).

The NHIA Act also provides for the development of a unique database, which is ICT driven, capable of warehousing all the data concerning health schemes in Nigeria, including those at the lower component units' level of the federation (local and state government levels). This will make it easy for the nation to gather the needed data concerning healthcare requirements of the general populace with a view to leveraging on the available resources to meet these envisage healthcare needs. One of the major advantages of the new Act is that all the states of the federation and the FCT will now establish health insurance agencies since it is now a requirement for all Nigerians. The creation of such an agency is a precondition to accessing the basic healthcare fund as stipulated in section 13 (8) of the Act. For proper coordination, firms are to register with the NHIA as health insurance service providers.

As for the contribution to the health scheme, this will come from employers and employees in the formal sector of the economy and also from individuals, families and groups in the informal sector as expressly stated in section 31(1) of the Act. For the extremely poor and vulnerable group of people who do not have the capacity to participate, section 31(2) submits that the three tiers of government (federal, state and local) shall intervene on their behalf. Section 47(1) addresses issues relating to litigation by unsatisfactory persons by arguing that 'No action shall lie against the authority and its agents' without writing at least one month before to the NHIA about such grievance. The composition of membership of the NHIA council is to be drawn from the federal and state health institutions and civil society groups, via certain criteria of eligibility. It remains to be seen if the NHIA will improve on the NHIS and by extension improve the existential health conditions of the average Nigerian. Will the NHIA radically increase the confidence of Nigerians in the nation's health institutions? Will it substantially reduce the brain drain in the health sector and end the incessant industrial actions therein? Only time can provide answers to these questions.

Conclusion

The inescapable verdict as it concerns the politics of healthcare reform in Nigeria is a bleak one, as most of the indices relating to healthcare in the nation are not on their optimal levels. To be sure the governance structure and behavioural trajectories of successive leaders have not helped. Furthermore, prolonged military rule, which had the unintended consequence of desecrating core federal principles, was oftentimes a major impediment to the emergence of well-constructed health sector reforms. This chapter deployed Michel Foucault's concept of biopower to examine the politics of healthcare reforms in Nigeria. One governance form through which this anomaly manifested was through the usurpation of the powers of the local governments. In a three-tier federal structure, the local government is the closest institution to the people, and it affords them the opportunity to have access to public facilities.

Health sector reforms, especially in the context of primary healthcare programmes, have suffered in part due to the fact that the central and component units have often been the major centres of power. While this tendency took root during the military era of the postcolonial history of the Nigerian state, it nevertheless became a permanent feature of Fourth Republic politics in Nigeria. Before now, the local government system in Nigeria continues to operate without autonomy. However, local governments are now empowered to receive direct allocation. However, the level of implementation is a far cry to the expected standard. The nation will have a better healthcare regime if these issues are checked in line with the devolution of power from the centre to the local government level.

References

Anaemene, B.U. (2016). Health Sector Reforms and Sustainable Development in Nigeria: A Historical Perspective. *Journal of Sustainable Development in Africa*, 18(4): 50–66.

Anaemene, B.U. and Aworawo, D. (2014). Indigenous Health Practices in Africa. In Osuntokun, J. (Ed.), *African Peoples, Cultures and Civilization* (pp. 77–85). Ede: Redeemer's University Press.

Aregbeshola, B.S. (2021). Towards Health System Strengthening: A Review of the Nigerian Health System From 1960 to 2019. *SSRN*, 14 January 2021. https://

ssrn.com/abstract=3766017; http://dx.doi.org/10.2139/ssrn.3766017. Accessed 17 June 2021.

Asuzu, M.C. (2004). The Necessity of a Health Systems Reform in Nigeria. *Journal of Community Medicine and Primary Health Care*, 16(1): 1–3.

Ball, S. (1998). Big Policies/Small World: An Introduction to International Perspectives in Education Policy. *Comparative Education*, 34(2): 119–129.

Burrows, M. and Engelke, P. (2020). *What World Post-Covid-19? Three Scenarios.* Washington, DC: Atlantic Council.

Campbell, T. and Sitze, A. (2013). *Biopolitics: A Reader.* Durham: Duke University Press.

Easton, D. (1965). *A Framework for Political Analysis.* Englewood Cliffs, NJ: Prentice-Hall Inc.

Edelman, M. (1988). *Constructing the Political Spectacle.* Chicago: University of Chicago Press.

Faleye, O.A. (2017). Environmental Change, Sanitation and Bubonic Plague in Lagos, 1924–31. *International Review of Environmental History*, 3(2): 89–103.

Faleye, O.A. (2023). COVID-19 Pandemic, Geopolitics of Health and Security Entanglement in West Africa. In Moyo, I. and Ndlovu-Gatsheri, S.J. (Eds.) *COVID-19 Pandemic and the Politics of Life.* London: Routledge.

Faleye, O.A. and Akande, T.M. (2019). Beyond "White Medicine": Bubonic Plague and Health Interventions in Colonial Lagos. *Gesnerus: Swiss Journal of the History of Medicine and Sciences*, 76(1): 90–110.

Fatunmole, M. (2022). Key Issues in Nigeria's New National Health Insurance Authority Act. www.icirnigeria.org/key-issues-in-new-national-health-insurance-authority-act.html. Accessed 6 August 2022.

Federal Government of Nigeria (FGN). (1970). *Second National Development Plan 1970–1974: Programme of Post-War Reconstruction and Development.* Lagos: Federal Government Press.

Federal Government of Nigeria (FGN). (1975). *Third National Development Plan, 1975–1980.* Lagos: Federal Government Press.

Federal Government of Nigeria (FGN). (2022). *The National Health Insurance Authority Act.* Abuja: Federal Government of Nigeria.

FMOH. (2004). *Health Sector Reform Programme: Thrusts with a Logical Framework and Plans of Action, 2004–2007.* Abuja: Federal Ministry of Health.

Fogel, R. (1991). The Conquest of High Mortality and Hunger in Europe and America: Timing and Mechanisms. In Higgonet, P., Landes, D., and Rosovsky, H. (Eds.) *Favourites of Fortune: Technology, Growth and Economic Development Since the Industrial Revolution* (pp. 33–71). Cambridge: Harvard University Press.

Gabriel, J.M. (2017). David Easton's "Authoritative Value Allocation" – Activating the Definition's Potential. *SSRN*, 1 February 2017. https://ssrn.com/abstract=2909910 or http://dx.doi.org/10.2139/ssrn.2909910.

Leftwich, A. (2008). *Developmental States, Effective States and Poverty Reduction: The Primacy of Politics.* Geneva: United Nations Research Institute for Social Development.

Muiu, M. (2002). Globalisation and Hegemony: Which Way Africa. *Journal of Policy Studies*, 8(1): 68–88.

Nwabuzor, E. and Mueller, M. (1985). *An Introduction to Political Science for African Students.* London: Macmillan.

Ogunbekun, I., Ogunbekun, A., and Orobatan, N. (1999). Private Health Care in Nigeria: Walking the Tightrope. *Health Policy and Planning*, 14(2): 174–178.

Olukoju, A. (2003). *Infrastructure Development and Urban Facilities in Lagos, 1861–2000*. Ibadan: IFRA.

Omoruan, A., Bamidele, A., and Philips, O. (2009). Social Health Insurance and Sustainable Health Care Reform in Nigeria. *Ethno-Med*, 3(2): 105–110.

Osaghae, E.E. (2002). *Crippled Giant: Nigeria Since Independence*. Ibadan: John Archers Publishers Ltd.

Popoola, D. (1993). Nigeria: Consequences for Health. In Aderanti, A. (Ed.) *The Impact of Structural Adjustment in Africa: Implications for Education, Health and Employment* (pp. 92–97). London: Heinemann.

Porta, M. (Ed.). (2014). *A Dictionary of Epidemiology* (6th Edition). New York: Oxford University Press.

Sinnerbrink, R. (2005). From Machenschaft to Biopolitics: A Genealogical Critique of Biopower. *Critical Horizons*, 6(1): 239–265.

Synge, R. (1993). *Nigeria: The Way Forward*. London: Euromoney Books.

Transparency International. (2021). Corruption Perception Index 2020. www.transparency.org/en/cpi. Accessed 19 June 2021.

UNICEF. (2000). *The Progress of Nations*. New York: The United Nations Children's Fund (UNICEF).

UNICEF. (2021). Nigeria: Key Demographic Indicators. www.data.unicef.org/country/nga.

Winslow. (1920). *Primary Health System in Nigeria*. Lagos, Nigeria: Elmore Publishers.

2 Framing Climate Change-Public Health Nexus in the Political Economy of Adaptive Systems in Postcolonial Africa

Olukayode A. Faleye, Tanimola M.
Akande, and Inocent Moyo

Introduction

The forces that shape history are unequal. The enduring inequality in accessing resources is reinforced by the politics and the political structure of society. Human extractive tendencies and the lack of harmony between nature and culture lead to conflicts between humans and the environment as well as between human groups whose existence depends on the ecosystem (Faleye, 2023). An important local response to environmental stress such as climate change is migration. Migration is driven by socio-economic and political factors. These factors are aggravated by environmental changes such as climate stress, stiffening economic insecurity due to inadequate water supply, and dwindling arable land for agriculture. These economic challenges manifest in restricted access to job opportunities and social services such as education and healthcare. Consequently, cross-border migration occurs as an extreme adaptive measure of livelihood resilience. The severity of climate stress is conditioned by the institutional structure of power which tends to further restrict access to scarce environmental resources through policy decisions that reinforce and justify domination (Wrathall et al., 2014).

The biopolitics of climate change is characterized by the political determinant of life and death in environmental policy. Biopolitics is the administration of life to determine the exercise and application of mortality through strategic policies targeting individuals (Foucault, 1976 [2003]). In this vein, the existence of institutions of state and their entitlement to legitimate force as a mark of sovereignty projects contemporary structures of political authority as arbiters of death in a necropolitical order that focuses on a target population rather than an individual (Mbembe, 2003). In postcolonial Africa, the necropolitical governance of death is legitimized by democratic institutions (Mbembe, 2019). Essentially, this is a democratization of death to sustain the uneven status quo in a post-truth world where the dominant powers in society reinforce their authority at the expense of "orderliness". Environmental stress and adaptation are accentuated by the power structures in society.

DOI: 10.4324/9781003429135-4

Therefore, this chapter frames the politics of climate stress, its manifestation in extractive violence, social conflicts, cross-border migration, and public health in Sub-Saharan Africa. Stated differently, the chapter examines the politics of climate change, socio-ecological conflicts, and their impact on public health in Sub-Saharan Africa by deploying the socio-ecological systemic approach which provides a deep understanding of the intertwined dynamics of social institutions and ecosystem complexities and resilience. This is "a system of people and nature" "where social and ecological systems are mutually dependent" in "mutual interactions" (Harrington et al., 2010: 2773; Thomas et al., 2012: 69; Fidel et al., 2014: 48). A central compass of socio-ecological knowledge is the idea of sustainable development (Colding and Barthel, 2019). Human interference with the ecosystem results in environmental changes and uneven allocation of resources.

Mapping Climate Change and Societies in Sub-Saharan Africa: An Overview

Climate change leads to high temperatures, melting glaciers, and floods. The United Nations regarded these features of climate change as products of "long-term shifts in temperatures and weather patterns" as a result of rare natural causes of solar transformation and volcanic eruptions as well as the socio-cultural activities of "burning fossil fuels" (United Nations, n.d.). These have a serious impact on human health, environmental health, food security, and disease control. Climate change could have a range of impacts on mental health due to the nature of exposure. This exposure includes natural disasters such as floods, hurricanes, and wildfires; drought and heat stress; sustained high temperatures; and rising sea levels (Palinkas and Wong, 2020). These climate issues reduce agricultural productivity and undermine food security, thereby deepening the level of poverty in society. Poverty limits access to social services, including education and healthcare. Food insecurity aggravates pre-existing ailments and stimulates the occurrence of non-existing ones like malnutrition.

The need for political intervention in climate change at the multilateral level engendered the United Nations' Sustainable Development Goals, Vision 2030. Vision 2030 fuses socio-economic and environmental issues into a wholesome public health framework (WHO, 2015). For instance, Goal 17, which points to the importance of sustainable production and consumption system with emphasis on the preference for clean energy, reveals the need for equity in the global production and distribution system in an indivisible natural world. This is an indictment on the capitalist unequal mode of production and distribution and an urgent need for an alternative sustainable system. Goal 12, which reflects on the importance of water supply and sanitation, envisions the importance of portable water in maintaining hygiene and preventing diseases such as cholera and kidney failure. Goal 13, which emphasizes the urgency of rolling back climate change, is interlocked with

Goal 14, which focuses on the conservation of marine resources. The abuse of marine resources through reckless extractive activities has a serious impact on climate change. Moreover, marine resources such as animals and plants play an important role in food security and serve as vital pharmaceutical materials for the treatment of diseases. Goal 15, with its emphasis on forest conservation, is aimed to reduce desiccation, and minimize loss of arable lands, and prevent the exposure of the human population to new strains of zoonotic diseases.

In Sub-Saharan Africa, environmental change impacts the system of production and public administration over time. The complexity of the exchange between the biological and physical elements of society negates any simplistic and monothetic environmental determinant of social evolution. As observed by Beinart (2000), the natural impact was often moderated by cultural knowledge, thereby rendering arguments that presuppose a pattern of livelihood determined by environmental conditionality simplistic. Nevertheless, extreme climatic changes impact cultures and could trigger unusual adaptation strategies with serious implications for the socio-political structure of societies. Colonialism is inherently a landmark in the climate history of Africa. It marked a significant cultural change in the usage of natural resources in the continent. Contrary to the capitalist venture, the African Indigenous Knowledge System emphasizes an intertwined survival of culture and nature which manifested in low-scale resource use and conservation.

However, colonial capitalism embraced large-scale resource use as a mark of technological advancement and economy of scale in an evolving global system built on uneven development. This colonial disruptive extraction undermines environmental health and livelihood in Sub-Saharan Africa. This necropolitical order undermines sustainable development and facilitated primitive accumulation to the detriment of global health. This is a political economy of death sustained by combined but uneven global development. Indeed, colonialism in Africa marked unprecedented ecological changes with implications for the environment. These environmental disasters found expression in epidemic outbreaks and pandemics in Sub-Saharan Africa during the colonial era (Kjekshus, 1977; Ngalamulume, 2006; Faleye, 2017). While the colonial system of exploitation was sustained in the postcolonial mode of production, the climatic effect of resource exploitation was more vivid in postcolonial Africa.

In Africa, climatic ideas of historical change have been traced to the drought of the 1960s, 1970s, and 1980s which significantly affected the arid parts of West Africa, East Africa, and Southern Africa (McCann, 1999). A significant impact of climate change has been felt by nomadic pastoralists with ensuing cross-border migration and cross-cultural conflicts in Sub-Saharan Africa (Olaniyan et al., 2021). The extant literature on climate change in Sub-Saharan Africa is built on environmental determinism with a focus on agricultural production, mobile cultures, and mining (Calzadilla et al., 2013; Coulibaly et al., 2020; Jahanger et al., 2022). In advancing this discourse, we ask the question: what is the impact of climatic change on public health in postcolonial Africa? We measure this climate change-public health nexus through the dynamics of local adaptive systems with reference to the political economy of natural resource extraction, food security, cross-border migration, and socio-ecological conflicts in postcolonial Africa.

Political Economy of Natural Resource Extraction, Climate Change, and Public Health in Postcolonial Africa

Climate change is a product of the global political economy due to the nature of natural resource extraction and usage in the international system. The huge contribution of Africa as the source of the vast quantity of energy resources in the metropolitan centres of great powers shows that any serious discourse on climate change should begin with the continent. The political forces that mould the African socio-ecological system are a dynamic in a web of global and local networks. While energy production is central to the discourse on climate change, African relevance in the global economy relates to the vast deposits of energy resources in the continent (DeBoom, 2021). Thus, the political economy of adaptive systems in Africa is embedded in the global and local networks of energy extraction, distribution, and its implication for the African people.

The impact of human activities on the climate is often measured by the trend of carbon-dioxide emissions. In this vein, Sub-Saharan Africa contributed only about 402,373 kt of CO_2 emissions in 1990. The African CO_2 emission witnessed a moderate rise over the following two decades. For instance, in 1995 the region emitted only 444,820 kt followed by 497,660 kt in 2000, 613,740 kt in 2005, 695,130 kt in 2010, 772,440 kt in 2015, and 823,770 kt in 2019. The African CO_2 emissions can be compared with some of the world's highest CO_2 emitters such as China, the United States, and the European Union (EU). The EU accounted for an all-time high CO_2 emission of 3,562,590 kt in 1990. This figure witnessed a gradual decline in the following two decades. In 1995, the EU CO_2 emission stood at 3,391,600 kt followed by about 3,362,380 kt in 2000, 3,488,150 kt in 2005, 3,213,190 kt in 2010, 2,895,700 kt in 2015 and 2,724,970 kt in 2019. The United States accounts for 4,844,520 kt in 1990, 5,117,040 kt in 1995, and a huge rise of 5,775,810 kt in 2000 followed by a steady but moderate decline of 5,753,490 kt in 2005, 5,392,110 in 2010, 4,990,710 kt in 2015 and 4,817,720 kt in 2019. China was responsible for a CO_2 emission of 2,173,360 kt in 1990 followed by a high rise of 3,088,620 kt in 1995, 3,346,530 kt in 2000 and 5,824,630 kt in 2005. The period between 2005 and 2010 was phenomenal as the Chinese CO_2 emission rose to a huge 8,474,920 kt in 2010, 9,861,100 kt in 2015, and 10,707,220 kt in 2019 (see Figure 2.1). In 2020, Africa contributed only 3.8% of global carbon dioxide emissions (Statista, 2022). Nevertheless, the continent is most affected by the deleterious effects of climate change.

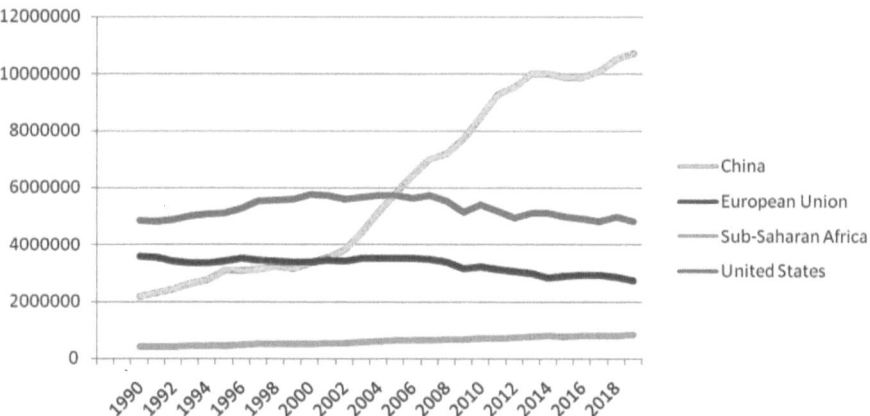

Figure 2.1 Climate Change by CO₂ Emissions (kt), Sub-Saharan Africa, European Union, United States and China, 1990–2019

Source: Authors' computation based on World Bank data on Climate Change by CO₂ Emissions (kt). https://data.worldbank.org/topic/climate-change?locations=ZG-EU-US-CN. Accessed 25 April 2023.

The variance in carbon-dioxide emissions in Figure 2.1 reflects the level of economic productivity of the countries in the context of manufacturing and international trade. This is indicated by their Gross Domestic Product (GDP) per capita Purchasing Power Parity (PPP) rate in the last two decades. Here, China's GDP by PPP in 1990 was 1.62 trillion. This was close to Sub-Saharan Africa's 1.51 trillion and far apart from the United States' account of 10.1 trillion and the EU's 11.99 trillion. In 2021, While Sub-Saharan Africa's underdeveloped GDP per PPP stood at 4.81 trillion, China accounted for 24.86 trillion, United States' GDP by PPP in the same year stood at 21.13 trillion and the EU accounted for 21.81 trillion (World Bank, 2023). These figures show that these countries' contribution to the global GDP is in tandem with the quantity of CO₂ emitted to justify economic productivity and growth.

Having created the foundation for its economic prosperity through the reckless extraction of fossil fuel from Sub-Saharan Africa, the Global North is set to consolidate this gain by moving towards green energy and technology. The question may be asked: can Africa leapfrog into economic development through green energy and technology? Can Africa afford the cost of the proposed green economic development plan? If Africa could not convert its cheap so-called "dirty" energy resources into economic prosperity, the green developmental proposal is like building a castle in the air. While the Global North moves towards a green economy, the level of underdevelopment in Africa coupled with the rise of alternative non-Western great powers such as China means that the survival of Africa is hinged on producing fossil fuel for the global energy market. Africa is home to the world's major deposit of both oil and solid minerals, and its economy depends largely on the international trade in primary goods such as petroleum and precious stones. In essence, African underdevelopment and the existence of markets for its fossil fuel means that the so-called "dirty" energy is not going away at the global level irrespective of the green multilateral agreements signed in the Global North. This will facilitate the speed of climate change and subsequently reverse the artificial capitalist gains in the long run. Indeed, contrary to the capitalist uneven mode of extraction and distribution, climate change is a leveller.

Climate change has the potential to reinforce social inequality by deepening the level of political irresponsibility, violent crisis, and human insecurity in postcolonial Africa. Beyond colonialism, "the sustenance of colonial institutions in the postcolonial era by the African political elites ensured the uninterrupted raping of the continent's human and natural resources" (Faleye, 2019: 82). This postcolonial catastrophe is reflective of the degenerative economic performance of most states in Sub-Saharan Africa. The diversion of public revenue into private pockets through the help of Western financial institutions amidst the absence of environmentally inclined sustainable investment means that the continent remains unprepared for climate change in a world clamouring for a transition from "dirty" to "clean" energy. Thus, deliberate investment must be made by the developed world to facilitate economic development in Africa. This is a necessary reparation for the age-old extractive violence in the continent; otherwise, the emerging climate Armageddon facilitated by global capitalism implies that we are all going under.

The clamour for green energy seems to have justified the extraction of certain solid minerals used as raw materials to produce clean energy. This is the legitimization of environmental degradation in Africa in the name of green energy sourcing. As noted by DeBoom (2021) Africa is one of the largest sources of mineral resources required to scale down climate change. For instance, while the Democratic Republic of the Congo accounts for 60% of the global production of cobalt used in battery production, Malawi is an emerging major global source of neodymium and praseodymium used in the manufacturing of wind turbines and electric vehicles. Whereas the mining and production of these raw materials are justified based on mitigating climate change through alternative energy sources such as electricity and wind, the African poor bear the socio-ecological cost. It is on this note that DeBoom (2021) asserts:

> There is both continuity and change in these distributive geographies. Extractive projects that undermine the sustainability of African political economies for the benefit of outside actors continue a long history of wealthier people and places outsourcing the negative externalities of accumulation and consumption to poorer people and places. Yet whereas "dirty" extractive endeavours have been rendered legitimate in the name of colonialism, nationalism, racial capitalism, or energy

security, among other justifications, "green" extractive projects are often justified in the name of universal climate salvation, including for the very populations most likely to bear their costs.

(p. 902)

The foregoing echoes Wrathall et al.'s (2014) assertion that climate stress reinforces pre-existing landscape of political domination and inequality. Using China's extraction of uranium from Namibia in Southern Africa as an example, DeBoom (2021) observed the sacrificial disposal of minority groups living around the uranium minefields of Erongo through livelihood disruption and gradual radiation exposure which in the long run could result in epidemic cancer and hereditary defects among the locals. This is particularly worrisome considering the externalization of uranium extraction to Africa despite the huge reserve of the same mineral in China. In this way, necropolitical extractive endeavours emanating from interests outside the continent are synonymous with a public policy that legitimizes death.

Climate Change-Induced-Cross-Border Migration, Socio-Ecological Conflicts and Public Health in Postcolonial Africa

African societies have often responded to climatic change and socio-political transformations through various adaptive measures that reflect the local political structure. The Nunu people, whose abode straddles the bank of Zaire and the Likwala aux Herbes Rivers, derived a lot of marine resources from seasonal flooding in most part of the year (Harms, 1988). Rather than being a curse, this environmental challenge ensured the breeding of many species of fish and a bounty harvest as the water fell. This was moderated by the dominant political group headed by the "Water Lords", who control the rich aquatic environment, thereby forcing a substantial section of the population to migrate elsewhere or diversify the nature of their livelihood. This shows that the dominant political structure in society impacts resource distribution and stimulates varieties of livelihood resilience in the face of climate stress. Climate change impacts food security in Sub-Saharan Africa. As noted by DeVries (1981), whereas a change in climate could impact a particular productive activity, the potency of cultural and adaptive response to climatic variability creates a complex causation of social change in the face of climatic instability. Here, an assessment of human adaptive responses to climatic change, food security, and cross-border migration unveils the socio-political outcome of the ecological transformation in Sub-Saharan Africa. This is the case of institutional moderation of resource use through the power that allocates and restricts access.

In Africa, a major feature of ecological conflicts is human insecurity where those displaced by drought and famine found succour in banditry. More than the mental manifestation of climate stress as depression in individuals, mental stress emanating from food insecurity and livelihood uncertainty in a population group often leads to violent conflicts as an adaptive response in Sub-Saharan Africa. Exclusive planning and bureaucratic corruption in the face of drought and food insecurity have been compounded by militia movements that seek alternative governance of the natural environment and societies in Mali, Nigeria, Somalia, and Sudan among others. The activities of al-Qaeda or the Islamic State in Mali, Boko Haram and bandits in Nigeria are an offshoot of environmental vulnerability and non-state response from militia groups who saw serious business in addressing local grievances against the state. Containing these socio-ecological conflicts is difficult due to the inability of political elites to bridge the complexities between the pure sciences and the social context. As Raineri (2020: 3) puts it:

> Environmental security policies in the Sahel are, by and large, shaped by policy, military and non-governmental organisation (NGO) actors who appear to see limited added value in the inputs of social science. As a result, climate change mitigation and environmental protection measures in the region have mostly failed to keep up with the standards of evidence-based policymaking. This neglect has paved the way to spectacular failures.

In the borderlands of Mali, Burkina Faso, and Niger in the Sahel, scientific studies attribute climate change to cultural practices that propel deforestation, thereby motivating policy interventions that undermine the survival of the poorest groups in society. The reduction of grazing land due to intensive farming that increased the production of food crops by elitist investors, insensitive environmental conservation policies that culminated in taxation on firewood collection, and restrictions on wildlife hunting amidst starvation at the population level fuel local resentment of political authorities (Raineri, 2020). Climate-induced food insecurity leads to nutritional deficiency and related health challenges in Sub-Saharan Africa. In the face of poor performance of governments and the tactical obliteration of target populations, the adaptive response is the diversification into banditry, terrorism, violent conflicts, and cross-border migration to other parts of West Africa, such as Nigeria, leading to a circle of violent conflicts between the migrants and their host communities.

The War in Darfur started in 2003 between an Arab-dominated government of Sudan and Darfur's non-Arab population over issues of social inequality and uneven resource distribution. Central to the issues were water supply and land use between nomadic (Arabs) and sedentary farming (Fur) populations. The root of the socio-ecological crisis can be traced to the colonial period when the British marginalized Darfur as punishment for the bitter war of conquest. This colonial pattern of social inequality was reinforced in the postcolonial era as considerable national resources were concentrated in the state capital Khartoum, inhabited by the elites. The severe drought of the 1980s witnessed the transformation of the Arab nomads of the semi-arid plains into a sedentary population seeking land resources in the fertile oasis of Darfur. One such place, Jebel Mara, was traditionally inhabited by local farmers, the *Fur* people. In the face of climate stress, the reinvigoration of uneven environmental policies such as the Unregistered Land Act of 1970, which places the non-registered land at the disposal of the state, made most of the black Sudanese in Darfur landless people (Abouyoub, 2012). The attempts of the nomadic Arabs to displace the black Sudanese with the tactical support of the Sudanese Arab government triggered a wave of unprecedented political violence since 2003.

Khartoum reinforced the existing social inequality with repressive violence and genocide as the marginalized resorted to insurgency as the last resort. As observed by De Juan (2015), the war was a product of long-term variations in water and vegetation distribution coupled with migration adaptive responses in a volatile region characterized by ethnic diversity which triggered fierce competition for resources. This is a circle of violent conflicts driven by environmental vulnerability emanating from environmental "necropolicies" (environmental policies of death) and the associated food insecurity and fatalities of a targeted population. The attendant blockages of transportation networks and raiding of ungoverned spaces by militia groups obstruct local peoples' access to health services in Sub-Saharan Africa. Climate-induced violent conflicts show that more than the direct effects of climate change, the social responses through the structure of power in society could determine who lives or dies in a time of environmental crisis.

Conclusion

This chapter unveils the nexus between climate stress, public health, and the socio-political structure of societies in Sub-Saharan Africa. It showcases the dynamics of climate change from the lenses of power asymmetry, uneven allocation of resources, and sustainable development in the region. Drawing useful insight from postcolonial theories of biopolitics and necropolitics, the chapter uncovers the complexities of climate change in the context of the political economy of adaptive systems in Sub-Saharan Africa. It reveals the connection between $-CO_2$ emission and the global political economy of development based on the trend analysis of economic indicators in some of the highest emitters of CO_2 in comparison to Africa. In this vein, the variances in CO_2 emissions reflect the economic productivity of the developed and emerging economies. The global political economy of development perpetuates Africa in the cycle of mineral extraction, socio-ecological conflicts, food insecurity, unstable cross-border migration, and obstruction to healthcare services. Nevertheless, the study suggests that Africa could be central to the reversal of climate change; however, deliberate investment must be made by the developed world to facilitate rapid economic development in Africa as a redress of the age-old extractive violence and its associated public health challenges.

References

Abouyoub, Y. (2012). The Forgotten Culprit: The Ecological Dimension of the Darfur Conflict. *Race, Gender and Class*, 19(1/2): 150–176.

Beinart, W. (2000). African History and Environmental History. *African Affairs*, 99(395): 269–302.

Calzadilla, A., Zhu, T., Rehdanz, K., Tol, R.S., and Ringler, C. (2013). Economywide Impacts of Climate Change on Agriculture in Sub-Saharan Africa. *Ecological Economics*, 93: 150–165.

Colding, J. and Barthel, S. (2019). Exploring the Social-Ecological Systems Discourse 20 Years Later. *Ecology and Society*, 24(1). https://doi.org/10.5751/ ES-10598-240102.

Coulibaly, T., Islam, M., and Managi, S. (2020). The Impacts of Climate Change and Natural Disasters on Agriculture in African Countries. *Economics of Disasters and Climate Change*, 4: 347–364.

De Juan, A. (2015). Long-term Environmental Change and Geographical Patterns of Violence in Dafur, 2003–2005. *Political Geography*, 45: 22–33.

DeBoom, M.J. (2021). Climate Necropolitics: Ecological Civilization and the Distributive Geographies of Extractive Violence in the Anthropocene. *Annals of the American Association of Geographers*, 111(3): 900–912. https://doi.org/10.1080/ 24694452.2020.1843995.

DeVries, J. (1981). Measuring the Impact of Climate on History: The Search for Appropriate Methodologies. In Rotberg, R. and Rabb, T. (Eds.), *Climate and History: An Interdisciplinary History*. Princeton: Princeton University Press.

Faleye, O.A. (2017). Environmental Change, Sanitation and Bubonic Plague in Lagos, 1924–31. *International Review of Environmental History*, 3(2): 89–103.

Faleye, O.A. (2019). Border Securitisation and Politics of State Policy in Nigeria, 2014–2017. *Insight on Africa*, 11(1): 78–93.

Faleye, O.A. (2023). COVID-19 Pandemic, Geopolitics of Health and Security Entanglement in West Africa. In Moyo, I. and Ndlovu-Gatsheri, S.J. (Eds.), *COVID-19 Pandemic and the Politics of Life*. London: Routledge.

Fidel, M., Kliskey, A., Alessa, L., and Sutton, O.P. (2014). Walrus Harvest Locations Reflect Adaptation: A Contribution from a Community-Based Observing Network in the Bering Sea. *Polar Geography*, 37(1): 48–68. http://dx.doi.org/10.1080/1088 937X.2013.879613.

Foucault, M. (1976 [2003]). *Society Must Be Defended: Lectures at the College de France, 1975–1976*. London: Allen Lane.

Harms, R. (1988). *Games Against Nature: An Eco-Cultural History of the Nunu of Equatorial Africa*. Cambridge: Cambridge University Press.

Harrington, R., Anton, C., Dawson, T.P., de Bello, F., Feld, C.K., Haslett, J.R., Kluvánkova-Oravská, T., Kontogianni, A., Lavorel, S., Luck, G.W., Rounsevell, M.D.A., Samways, M.J., Settele, J., Skourtos, M., Spangenberg, J.H., Vandewalle, M., Zobel, M., and Harrison, P.A. (2010). Ecosystem Services and Biodiversity Conservation: Concepts and a Glossary. *Biodiversity and Conservation*, 19(10): 2773–2790. http://dx.doi.org/10.1007/s10531-010-9834-9.

Jahanger, A., Usman, M., Murshed, M., Mahmood, H., and Balsalobre-Lorente, D. (2022). The Linkages between Natural Resources, Human Capital, Globalization, Economic Growth, Financial Development, and Ecological Footprint: The

Moderating Role of Technological Innovations. *Resources Policy*, 76(102569). https://doi.org/10.1016/j.resourpol.2022.102569.

Kjekshus, H. (1977). *Ecology Control and Economic Development in East African History*. London: Heinemann.

Mbembe, J.A. (2003). Necropolitics. *Public Culture*, 15(1): 11–40.

Mbembe, J.A. (2019). *Necropolitics*. Durham: Duke University Press.

McCann, J.C. (1999). Climate and Causation in African History. *The International Journal of African Historical Studies*, 32(2/3): 261–279.

Ngalamulume, K. (2006). Plague and Violence in Saint-Louis-du-Sénégal, 1917–1920. *Cahiers d'études africaines*, 183. https://doi.org/10.4000/etudesafricaines.6027.

Olaniyan, R., Faleye, O.A., and Moyo, I. (Eds.). (2021). *Transborder Pastoral Nomadism and Human Security in Africa: Focus on West Africa*. London: Routledge.

Palinkas, L.A. and Wong, M. (2020). Global Climate Change and Mental Health. *Current Opinion in Psychology*, 32: 12–16.

Raineri, L. (2020). Sahel Climate Conflicts? When (Fighting) Climate Change Fuels Terrorism. *European Union Institute for Security Studies, Brief*, 20: 1–8. www.jstor.org/stable/resrep28786. Accessed 25 April 2023.

Statista. (2022). Africa's Share in Global Carbon Dioxide (CO_2) Emissions from 2000 to 2021. https://www.statista.com/statistics/1287508/africa-share-in-global-co2-emissions/. Accessed 18 July 2023.

Thomas, C.R., Gordon, I.J., Wooldridge, S., and Marshall, P. (2012). Balancing the Tradeoffs between Ecological and Economic Risks for the Great Barrier Reef: A Pragmatic Conceptual Framework. *Human and Ecological Risk Assessment*, 18(1): 69–91. http://dx.doi.org/10.1080/10807039.2012.631470.

United Nations. (n.d.). What Is Climate Change. *Climate Action. . . .*? Accessed 24 April 2023.

World Bank. (2023). GDP by Purchasing Power Parity: Sub-Saharan Africa, European Union, United States and China, 1990–2021 (Constant 2017 International $). *World Bank's World Development Indicators Database*. https://data.worldbank.org/indicator/NY.GDP.MKTP.CD? Accessed 26 April 2023.

World Health Organization. (2015). *Transforming Our World: The 2030 Agenda for Sustainable Development*. Geneva: World Health Organization. https://sustainabledevelopment.un.org/post2015/transformingourworld. Accessed 24 April 2023.

Wrathall, D.J., Bury, J., Carey, M., Mark, B., McKenzie, J., Young, K., Baraer, M., French, A., and Rampini, C. (2014). Migration amidst Climate Rigidity Traps: Resource Politics and Social-Ecological Possibilism in Honduras and Peru. *Annals of the Association of American Geographers*, 104(2): 292–304.

3 Rhetoric of Public Policies and Equity in Access to Healthcare in Postcolonial Senegal

Marième Ciss

Introduction

This chapter examines the socio-political dimension of public policy with a focus on health inequalities in postcolonial Senegal. In a global context, scholars have sought to analyse the process of highlighting social inequalities in health in the world and agree on the idea that the growth of these inequalities is the result of several factors including the governance of state, industrialization, liberalism, capitalism, and urbanization. In this regard, health inequalities have been explained from the context of complex mechanisms and multiple actions in which economic liberalism and the shrinking of the role of the state are determining factors (Rainhorn, 2001). As observed by Fassin (1996) human societies have gone from "the inscription on the body" – in the form of wounds, traces or marks of torture, wear and tear at work, etc. – from the social hierarchy to "the incorporation of inequalities", that is to say, the inscription in bodies of social inequalities in the form of disparities in the face of illness and death. Indeed, "if in all societies the social order is transcribed in the body, this transcription has not always taken place in the form of disparities in the face of illness and death" (Fassin, 1996: 38). In traditional societies, the social order was not expressed on bodies in the form of differential mortality and morbidity according to status or social class to which they belong. It resulted more in relationships of domination that could manifest themselves in physical violence.

It is therefore the process of social differentiation, urbanization, industrialization, and globalization which has transformed the relations of production and relations with the environment. The hierarchical structure of the social order began to express itself in the bodies in the form of disparities in life expectancy, attrition at work, and morbidity. The power architecture of the state holds the monopoly of legitimate physical violence and decides the manner of the expression of violence on bodies. As observed by Mbembe (2003, 2019) this exercise of the power to decide who lives or dies is indicated in the idea of necropolitics. Thus, there is disparity in the severity of illness or diseases based on the nature of power relations in society.

DOI: 10.4324/9781003429135-5

In this vein, the character of the social structure and materialism conditions the production of health inequalities (Aaich, 2004). Thus, the legitimization of death is often expressed through the nexus of health inequalities and risk behaviours, thereby the social structure of health inequality, by blaming the dead for their death. The amplification effect resides in the fact that when a new unfavourable event or a risk factor appears, it increases inequalities between social groups. As for the effect of increasing and maintaining inequalities, it is linked to the socially acquired differential disposition to the appropriation of existing resources and knowledge in terms of prevention and care. In Africa, health policies have accentuated the marginalization of certain already very vulnerable sub-groups in favour of a greater financial viability of health facilities. As noted by Ridde and Girard (2004) exemption from payment for the indigent is a viable solution, but it is not socially feasible.

In Senegal, there is limitation of public action in the quest for greater equity in terms of access to healthcare. Thus, "faced with the obstacles encountered by the poor and their exclusion from health care systems, it is important today to affirm more strongly than ever the right to life and health" (Becker et al., 2008: 106). In this vein, Fall and Ndoye noted the greater division between urban and rural areas, on the one hand, and between areas polarized by a health structure and non-polarized areas, on the other hand. The structural disparity in the implementation of health policies creates inequalities between territories. As observed by Faye (2008), Senegalese health has failed in the care of local people due to widespread inequality in the structure of health infrastructure.

While studies have documented the challenges surrounding inequalities in access to healthcare, the extant literature has not sufficiently shown why health equity policies are still excluded from the health system despite the persistence of rhetoric tending to make visible the need to combat inequalities. It is against this backdrop that this chapter examines the nature of the relationship between the rhetoric of equity in public health policy and its translation into practice in Senegal.

Conceptual Note

Institutions and laws, however effective, must be reformed or abolished if they are unjust. The idea of "unjust inequalities" reflects on the politically and socially avoidable inequalities. In this respect, it is worth recalling that one of the founding principles of the state is to counteract social inequalities by promoting measures of solidarity and redistribution of resources. This social role of the state is one of the major foundations of its legitimacy. Both national and international public health policies claim the obligation of equity and social justice as a guiding principle. All societies are hierarchically organized into age groups, gender, and economic and political statuses

(Fassin, 2000). Thus, whether it is related to wealth, work, health, education, or others, perfect equality has never been verified in the history of humanity. What remains is that the resources of the world, of a country, or of a region are unequally distributed. Seen in this light, health inequalities could be understood as a simple reflection of the hierarchical nature of any human society. However, a more detailed analysis suggests that the political and social factors have a considerable impact on these inequalities. Inequalities in the face of illness and death reveal the necropolitics that determines life and death in societies.

These inequalities manifest between developed and underdeveloped countries, between migrants and citizens, between urban and rural populations, between poor and rich in the same country, city, or neighbourhood. The 2003 WHO's health report reveals that in Africa there are 160 deaths per 1000 births, while in America and Northern Europe the figures are 22 and 19 per 1000 respectively, while the world average is around 80 deaths per 1000 births.

While life expectancy is around 80 years in developed countries, particularly in Europe, the United States, and Japan, it does not exceed 50 years in Third World countries. While disability-free life expectancy in the European Union increases by one year every four or five years, it is gradually decreasing in many Third World countries. Among the indicators of these inequalities between the North and the South, it can be noted, for example, that people living with HIV/AIDS in developed countries enjoy a longer life expectancy than those living in the Third World, thanks to more favourable social conditions and easier access to care. The examination of other indicators, such as the level of technical facilities, the distance to the nearest healthcare structure, material resources, the number of doctors, midwives, and nurses per inhabitant, further shows the extent of the health disparities between Western and Third World countries. Thus, it is now widely accepted that the determinants of health exist beyond the sphere of health and healthcare systems in the strict sense, and that these determinants are both social and political. Awareness of the unfair nature of health inequalities has led to major social policies in most European countries. The democratization of access to health services and the establishment of an accessible health insurance and social protection system in several European countries are part of this process.

As far as Sub-Saharan Africa is concerned, national and international public policies have had as their main argument the urgency of taking into account the equity dimension of access to healthcare. In Senegal, considering equity is more akin to justifying rhetoric that helps to mask persistent inequalities. Indeed, its permanence in the justification of current policies contrasts largely with the reality of the facts, but as Didier Fassin has so well shown that

> health policies, like any collective activity, have their myths that tell us their foundations. The narratives through which the authorised versions

of these myths are transmitted thus reveal the intention and the meaning that, more or less consciously, these policies are intended to give.

(Fassin, 2000: 213)

Jobert's model of political non-decision guides this study. As observed by Jobert (1985, 1992), non-decision does not mean the prevention of politicization of a problem through the justification and legitimization of government inaction. As Jobert noted:

> by non-decision we do not mean phenomena of total repression of the demands of certain social groups from the political arena, but situations where a new action or situation is recognised as necessary in the political discourse but no measures are taken to implement it.
>
> (Jobert, 1992: 224–225)

From the foregoing, we understand the non-decision model is an effective methodological alternative because it makes it possible to overcome one of the main impasses faced by public policy analysts: the fact that the objectives stated by decision-makers rarely correspond to the real aim of their actions. Being able to distinguish between rhetoric that justifies and rhetoric that structures – that is, rhetoric that actually informs public action – is one of the major challenges facing the public policy specialist. Referential are on the one hand a set of beliefs, representations, and techniques that structure the public policy scene. On the other hand, they constitute a set of tried-and-tested recipes, concrete solutions, and the substitute for explicit rules responsible for solving problems that have not yet been resolved. The referential approach shows the important role of public policy referential in the governability of societies and in the strengthening of the state function of maintaining social cohesion. Indeed, the interest and success of public policy referential depend on their ability to identify with dominant social values. Moreover, this conformity to values facilitates the creation and maintenance of the consensus and legitimization necessary for any public action. As observed by Jobert (1992), if Western societies have so far succeeded in averting crises, it is because they have been capable of intellectual learning in a constantly changing context. The permanent learning of the values to be reactivated to legitimize or justify public action is thus a prerequisite for the actors of the decision.

Assessing Health Equity in Senegal: Fairness Tested by the Facts

Postcolonial Senegal has put in place an important legal and institutional system for health coverage for the poor or "indigent", but the effectiveness of this system is poor. Indeed, there are considerable disparities in access to healthcare according to professional situation, and beyond these disparities there is a paradox: people with regular incomes and relatively capable of taking care of themselves are the privileged ones in the social protection system as well as the health insurance programme. In reality, most of the Senegalese population does not have access to medical coverage. In this regard, the DHS MICS 2010 reveals that overall; the majority of men and women surveyed have no medical coverage. Indeed, the percentages of women and men who do not have medical coverage are 94% and 92% respectively. These proportions are very high regardless of the socio-demographic characteristics of the women and men surveyed (DHS MICS, 2010–2011: 85).

Among the mechanisms for promoting equity in Senegal, at the lowest level of the health pyramid, are the health development committees (post and health centre), the hospital social services at the highest level, the IPRES, the Sesame plan, and recently the universal health coverage programme or CMU. In Senegal, a memo from the Ministry of Health reminds health managers of health posts and centres of a provision of the national guide of the health committee, which requires them to set aside 10% of their budget for the care of social cases. This measure should make it possible to counter the risk of exclusion generated by the application of the principle of cost recovery by users. Nevertheless, this system is not well integrated into the day-to-day work of health structures. Budgetary deficits, the heavy financial burden placed on the committees, ignorance of this system by the population, rationing strategies by those in charge, and difficulties linked to the criteria for identifying those entitled to benefits are all factors that explain this situation. Given their limited resources, the health committees cannot spend certain amounts on the care of the indigent. Moreover, the fear of an announcement effect and a possible explosion in demand means that this scheme is not popularized: "We are not going to propagate this possibility to the population; otherwise the health post will go bankrupt", an administrator in a healthcare facility told me.

Beyond the lack of information and insufficient resources, there are also cultural factors that lead some poor patients not to seek help even if they need it. "People here are so proud that they are not used to asking for help, it's not because there is a lack of social cases, but these people don't come out of pride", says a health committee chairman. Furthermore, the identification of social cases is also problematic, because even though poverty or indigence is supposed to be the main criterion for being covered by the committee, it is often very difficult to estimate the level of indigence of the patient. The decision to grant an exemption sometimes depends on the nature of the relationship between the managers and the patient. At this level, the role of the service providers is decisive, especially since they are the ones who are in direct contact with the patients. "It is the nurse who identifies the social cases, he tells me to consider them as social cases, and in the evening, when the payment is made to the treasurer, I tell him about it", says a ticket seller.

The role of community personnel (drug dealers, matrons, and community health workers) in the management of these social cases should not be over-looked, as the following words testify to the important role they play in this area: "the CHWs and matrons help me to identify social cases because they live with the people", said one PCI. This method of identifying social cases can be effective because matrons and community health workers (CHWs), while being part of the health staff, are opinion leaders who play a signifi-cant role in the management of community affairs, particularly in the area of health. Thus, they act as intermediaries between state personnel (ICP, doctor, midwife, etc.) and the community. In the absence of formal rules, cronyism, neighbourliness, and kinship tend to take precedence over the requirement of equity. In the context of poverty, the identification of the "indigent" has always been a problem for these types of social action. Despite the low level of income of the population, the unpredictable nature of illness, and the lack of health insurance, the committees are still struggling to fulfil their mission of assisting social cases. The management of "social cases" by the health committees suffers from this lack of formalization, cultural factors, insuf-ficient resources, and a failure to define priorities.

On the part of those in charge of health structures and health committees, the fear of the risks of bankruptcy is perceptible through the various inter-views with the actors concerned, and as a result, economic rationality tends to take precedence over considerations of equity. Faced with the need for effi-ciency, those in charge are more concerned with bailing out their funds than with caring for patients who are not solvent. As a result, they put more effort into investing in the productivity and competitiveness of their structures than in implementing the equity dimension of access to care. The regulation of 26 March 1962 on certificates of indigence in Senegal allows the "indigent" to obtain exemption from the costs of care in health services. Thus, there are social services in hospitals and certain health centres whose main function is to provide psychological and financial assistance to destitute and insolvent people. They can thus in principle benefit from total or partial exemption on the cost of consultation tickets, examinations, surgical interventions, etc. The case study of a mother found in a health centre gives an idea of the role of social services in the accessibility of healthcare to disadvantaged people as illustrated in the T.N. Case Studies, Sesame Plan, and the Universal Health Coverage in postcolonial Senegal.

T.N. Case Studies

With the permission of the person in charge of the care service, I contacted T.N. (34 years old), who was at the bedside of her 8-year-old child suffering from malaria and hospitalized. Married at the age of 20, T.N. is the mother of six children, two of whom have died, one of whom is in the care of her mother, and the other three live with her. Before her marriage, she used to go to Dakar to work as a domestic staff. Since her marriage, she has been doing laundry for others to support herself, but she tells us that it is an activity she cannot do full time, because she has children. According to the respondent:

> I brought him and he was detained. I had no money to bring him on Saturday, a neighbour lent me 5000f, I took a taxi and brought him to the Mbour 2 dispensary and they referred me there. I told them at the beginning to release us because I do not have enough to pay but when I was leaving, one of the agents called me to tell me that they would help me. They help us but sometimes we buy anyway . . . When a child has malaria, sometimes we have money to take him to hospital, some-times we don't, in which case we give him paracetamol. . . . If a child is ill and I don't have money to take him, I entrust myself to God.

T.N. had taken the trouble to call his mother to inform her of the situa-tion. This is how she left her village of origin to come and lend a helping hand: "She borrowed money and she came with that, we manage". Access to healthcare is therefore a real problem for this mother and her children:

> Three months ago I had a throat problem, there was a lump, I went to the pharmacy and they sold me a medicine that cost 3000f when I took it, it was useless, I stayed for a while and the signs went away. I had borrowed the 3000f from a lady, a neighbour, I did the laundry for her and she deducted her 3000f. . . . I didn't know that there was a social service that took care of the sick in hospitals.

All this reflects the difficulties poor households face in accessing healthcare and the strategies they use to access healthcare despite the challenges. This case shows the considerable support of the grandmother who came with the little money she had borrowed to stay with her daughter at the bedside of her granddaughter in the hospital.

These comments further confirm the importance of taking into account the financial barrier in accessing health services in postcolonial Senegal. The case of this mother shows the importance of social action in health struc-tures. When she arrived at the hospital, T.N. immediately wanted to return with her sick child because she knew she could not afford to pay the hospital bills. Nevertheless, thanks to a health worker found on the spot, she was able to access assistance from the social service. It can therefore be said that because of this service, an 8-year-old child was saved from a possible death from malaria. However, what is also important in this case is the lack of information and the absence of a guarantee against the risk of illness, which leads the poor person to refuse modern healthcare, even if it is necessary. How many patients delay seeking care or give it up simply because of these financial reasons? A health policy such as this makes the poor vulnerable to health challenges. In a way, it regulates the chances of who lives or dies in line with the economic status and social hierarchy of the patients. In an interview, the lead doctor of the health centre put the problem in these terms:

The third-party payer cannot be the individual who suffers; we cannot wait until he is ill to ask him to pay. Equity is quite possible in access to care, but provided that the state has this notion in mind so that the billionaire has the same chance of survival as the peasant, provided that it is a notion supported by the state.

(Health centre director)

This provider believes that the introduction of taxes on large companies and the informal sector (which take advantage of state privileges) can contribute to the implementation of equity in access to care. In the absence of third-party payment, it is difficult to guarantee an equitable health system, especially as the population alone is unable to meet the cost of their healthcare needs: "I still believe that the populace should not be left to their own devices, funds must be drawn from somewhere", the chief doctor insists. In a situation where the majority of the people are poor, on what basis can it be decided to provide healthcare services free of charge to some and refuse them to others. In principle, social service managers usually limit themselves to a short office interview, which sometimes leaves room for subjectivity. In addition, even if these enquiries are made, it is sometimes very difficult to determine the precise economic situation of the patient. Thus, it is common to see cases of refusal of care for purely subjective reasons.

In addition, like the health committees, access to the social service is compromised by the low level of information among those entitled to it: "People don't know that there is a social service at the hospital, sometimes it is me who informs them. They are not used to going out", disclosed one ICP interviewed in a village. Nevertheless, at this level, it seems that there is also a sort of strategy of withholding information on the existence of the social service and its main function. Still, as we have already seen with the health committees, the existence of hospital social services is unknown to the public. If there is one lack of equity that is rarely mentioned, it is the lack of information and orientation of the poor in health structures. This reality is illustrated by the saying "Hospital ku amul xalis doo Faju" (In hospital, if you do not have money, you don't get care) – often heard from patients.

Measures of Free or Exempted Payment: The Case of the Sesame Plan

In Senegal, medical health insurance for the elderly is a major challenge for the political authorities, given the generally precarious state of health of this social category, its generally low economic power, and the weakness of the social protection system. It is in this sense that the slogan "towards a society for all ages and without social exclusion" was conceived to promote the consideration of this segment of the population. The elderly represent a significant proportion of the Senegalese population and, until 2006, only 30% of this social category, that is, the beneficiaries of the IPRES and the FNR, had medical insurance, leaving the majority of these people without care.

It was in this context of poor coverage that the Sesame Plan was put in place. On 3 April 2006, during his traditional declaration to the nation on the eve of Independence Day, President Abdoulaye Wade announced the introduction of a specific form of health insurance for the elderly, the Sesame Plan:

> As you know, I have decided to grant free medicines to the elderly. This act reflects the ideal of inter-generational solidarity so characteristic of our people. . . . This is why I have instructed the Minister of Health and Disease Prevention to devise, with partners such as the Senegalese Pension Institute (IPRES); the National Pension Fund (FNR); the Dakar Faculty of Medicine and local authorities, a plan for medical insurance. It will enable the elderly to benefit from free care in selected hospitals, centres and health posts throughout the national territory.
>
> (Speech to the Nation, 3 April 2006)

The foregoing political decision was formulated to provide free care and medication for the elderly at all levels of the health pyramid. To this end, a subsidy of 700 million CFA francs from the state's own funds was initially earmarked to finance the plan. In its formulation, the Sesame Plan was supposed to ensure the generalization of medical coverage and access to medicines for all people aged 60 and above. However, were the stated ambitions the reflection of a well-developed political decision or were they rather, as some believe, a ruse to defuse the real or supposed reluctance of the elderly to support candidate Wade?

In its implementation, the package of services offered is very sparse or even non-existent in some health structures. Second, the reimbursement of the costs of services linked to the Sesame Plan is very problematic, as it is delayed and not complete. "The state owes us money for medicines, the reimbursements do not come. We cannot continue to give medicines otherwise we risk going bankrupt", said a card issuer in a health centre. At the central level, particularly at the Ministry of Health, this statement is not denied: "the rate of health insurance has decreased, and the files are arriving slowly because some hospitals have suspended insurance package due to lack of reimbursement by the state" (Sesame Plan focal person).

Those entitled to the scheme are disappointed, as the ambitions declared through the sesame are in stark contrast to the nature of the services offered. We know how great the hope raised by the speech of 3 April 2006 was, but this hope quickly dissipated and the words of this elderly person interviewed in a village speak volumes about this disappointment: "Anyone who wants to wait for the sesame to treat himself risks dying". If in the rhetoric one magnifies this initiative, one speaks of free care and medication for all elderly people in Senegal, the reality is different. The free care advocated in this initiative is less a reality than a rhetorical justification. The idea of the sesame was hailed for its ethical and social character, for the originality and innovation that it represented in the history of the health and social protection system in Senegal and, beyond, in Africa, but its implementation is far from what the political discourse says it is.

Universal Health Coverage: The Persistence of a 'Non-Decision' Policy

On 20 September 2013, President Macky Sall presided over the official launch of Universal Health Coverage (UHC) in Dakar. On that occasion, he announced his decision to make healthcare "free" for children under the age of five: "I have taken the decision to make healthcare free for children under the age of five and I ask the Minister of Health and Social Action to take all the necessary measures for its effective application from 1 October 2013". As soon as it was announced, the UHC, which was one of the president's electioneering promises, aroused a lot of hope and enthusiasm on the part of citizens, and its beginning was crowned by the provision of 5 billion CFA francs, including 1.7 billion CFA francs for mutual health insurance. The implementation of it was done gradually. It was initially intended to cover consultation, hospitalization, and vaccination costs in basic (health posts) and intermediate (health centres) structures. In addition, from 2014, all services offered in health posts and centres are declared free of charge.

As for hospital care, free access only concerns emergency care, which leads us to question the relevance of the term "free" in the qualification of this measure. Indeed, hospital care is the most difficult for households. This "free" measure was initially carried out in two phases: at the beginning, it was only the consultation fees (generally fixed at 200 CFA francs for children) which was free, and gradually all the other elements of the package of services offered in the health posts and centres were integrated. Beyond the lack of follow-up to this measure, the term "Universal Health Coverage" in its entirety seems inappropriate insofar as the vast majority of the population is still left out. How else can one explain the lack of political will regarding the need to strengthen the "Sesame Plan" for the elderly? All this justifies and confirms the predominance of the policy of "non-decision" which characterizes health equity policies. In fact, depending on the year, the same realities are designated by new words, slogans, and even new rhetoric, whereas in practice the terms ("Health for all", "For a society of all ages and without discrimination", "Universal health coverage", etc.) correspond very little to what the decision-makers actually do but rather constitute a social strategy for legitimization of political office.

Conclusion

This chapter shows that public policies relating to equity, as they manifest themselves in the daily reality of the healthcare system, have a very limited effectiveness and contrast with the rhetoric used to designate them in postcolonial Senegal. This rhetoric is certainly a very effective instrument for masking the failure of the state to fulfil its function of social protection of the populace. The analysis of the role of health committees, social hospital services, and free healthcare policies, including the Sesame Plan and the UHC, has highlighted the large gap that still needs to be filled to promote equity in access to healthcare. In reality, the emphases on the financial and political dimensions and the quest for efficiency have only favoured the inaccessibility of healthcare to the poorest. This implies a necropolitics of health services that condemn the poor to the grave in postcolonial Senegal.

References

Aaich, P. (2004). Processus cumulatif d'inégalités, effetsd'amplification et disposition à l'appropriation sociale. *Santé société et solidarité*, 2.

Becker, C., Diakhaté, M., and Fall, A. (2008). Répartition des ressources et équité dans l'accès à la santé: une reproduction des inégalités. In Daffé, G. and Diagne, A. (dir.) *Le Sénégal face aux défis de la pauvreté. Les oubliés de la croissance* (pp. 81–108). Dakar: Karthala, CRES and CREPOS.

Brunet-Jailly, J. (1993). Quel financement pour quels services de santé? In *Argent et Santé: expériences de financement communautaire en Afrique* (pp. 221–256). Paris: Actes du séminaire international.

Fassin, D. (1996). *L'espace politique de la santé: Essai de généalogie*. Paris: PUF.

Fassin, D. (2000). *Les enjeux politiques de la santé*. Paris: Karthala.

Faye, S.-L. (2008). Devenir mère au Sénégal: des expériences de maternité entre inégalités sociales et défaillances des services de soins. *cahiers santé*, 18(3).

Jobert, B. (1985). L'Étaten action. L'apport des politiques publiques. *Revue française de science politique*, 35(4): 654–682.

Jobert, B. (1992). Représentations sociales, controverses et débats dans la conduite des politiques publiques. *Revue française de science politique*, 42(2): 219–234.

Mbembe, J.A. (2003). Necropolitics. *Public Culture*, 15(1): 11–40.

Mbembe, J.A. (2019). *Necropolitics*. Durham: Duke University Press.

Rainhorn, J.-D. (2001). Un avenir incertain. In Rainhorn, J.-D. and Burnier, M.J. (dir.) *La santé au risque du marché: incertitudes à l'aube du XXIe siècle* (pp. 11–35). Paris: PUF.

Ridde, V. and Girard, J.-E. (2004). Douzeans après l'initiative de Bamako: constats et implications politiques pour l'équitéd'accès aux services de santé des indigents africains. *Santé publique*, 41: 37–51.

Wade, A. (2006). "Speech to the Nation", 3 April.

4 Spatial Politics of Health and the Control of Viral Hemorrhagic Fevers in Postcolonial Africa

Lessons from Lagos

Olukayode A. Faleye, Arthur C. Okafor, and Jonathan Dangana

Introduction

This study examines the nexus between demographic structure and health governance in Sub-Saharan Africa. Particular attention is directed to the nature of rural-urban migration and its implication for disease control in the region. Here, the focus is the endemiology of viral hemorrhagic fevers, including Lassa fever and Ebola virus disease (EVD), in Sub-Saharan Africa. The extant literature emphasizes the importance of demographic data in planning logistics for health intervention. Indeed, the analysis of age variances, ethnicity, and class and the transformation of the composite statistics through birth rate, death rate, and migration provide insight into the social determinants of population health. Demographic change impacts the structure of society and requires systemic control. The inherent relations between demographic structure, space, and governance create a political space of life and death (Faleye, 2023). This is engraved in the access to social services and infrastructure. Urbanization showcases the importance of contemporary demographic changes, infrastructure, and governance to population health (Connolly et al., 2021).

In the age of globalization, improved global transportation infrastructure and rural-urban migration facilitate the rapid growth of urban spaces as hubs of the emerging global society. As a result, the urban centers enjoy the political goodwill for infrastructural intervention than the rural areas. To this end, scholars have justified the vitality of the urban demography to global health and public health preparedness (Carter-Pokras et al., 2007; Allen and Katz, 2010). This is particularly true in developing societies in Sub-Saharan Africa where the rapid growth of population is more obvious in cities such as Lagos, Nigeria. The prioritization of urban centers in global development plan has led to rural-urban inequality with implications for disease control. The study of biopolitics and necropolitcs in the works of Michel Foucault and Achelle Mbembe unveils the political engineering of life and death in reference to target individuals or a population group in society (Foucault, 1982; Mbembe, 2003, 2019). This pattern of rural-urban inequality and spatial disparity in

DOI: 10.4324/9781003429135-6

resource distribution and health infrastructure legitimizes death in the rural areas. This is spatial necropolitics where demographic structure determines the expendability of a population. Moreover, the variability of disease environments implies the need for a unified equitable health intervention based on the peculiarity of a population need. Moreover, the rural environment is susceptible to viral hemorrhagic fevers (VHF) due to deforestation brought about by agricultural activities and the associated exposure to wildlife. The chapter answers the questions: what are the health implications of this spatial inequality between urban and rural areas in Sub-Saharan Africa? How does this spatial pattern of health intervention impact the endemiology Lassa Fever and EVD in the region?

Endemiology of Viral Hemorrhagic Fevers in Sub-Saharan Africa: An Overview

Viral hemorrhagic fevers are products of the environmental and socio-economic production system of rural communities. We examine two of the diseases in this category, that is, Lassa fever and Ebola virus disease (EVD). Lassa fever (LF) is a viral zoonotic disease spread by rodent – *Mastomysnatalensis* rats. It was first discovered in Nigeria in 1969 (Walker et al., 1982). The co-existence of other endemic diseases such as malaria and typhoid with Lassa fever poses a major challenge to the timely diagnosis of the latter. This is particularly the case of common symptoms shared by these tropical diseases such as fever, joint and abdominal pains, vomiting, and diarrhea among others. While Ribavirin is commonly deployed in the treatment of Lassa fever, the effectiveness of the drug administration is subject to the ability to diagnose the disease early in the affected patients (Happi et al., 2019). The chances of early diagnoses depend on the surveillance system on the ground. The LF disease pathology provides a path to its containment. Its animal reservoir is the *Mastomysnatalensis* rat found in many neighborhoods characterized by poor housing, dysfunctional sewerage, and refuse disposal common in rural areas and suburban locations in Nigeria. Hence, Lassa fever is a disease of underdevelopment and poverty.

The outbreak of Lassa fever in West African rural areas has been linked to cultural and environmental practices in the production of food such as Cassava flakes and the open-drying methods as well as local practices of consuming rats as delicacies. Clinical studies of LF morbidity and mortality are often based on data derived from the experiences of LF in rural areas. The mortality rate is higher among the older patients with an increase of about a 25% mortality risk for every ten years of age. The occurrence of LF among all age groups and occupational and gender divide is indicated. However, the infection is proportionally higher among school children, and the disease often leaves its mark on surviving victims which may include hearing issues (Asogun et al., 2012).

The acute viral hemorrahgic fever called Lassa fever, an arenavirus with non-specific symptoms (CDC, 2004), is known to have demonstrated a geometric trend in West African countries, with high incidence and fatality cases in recent years. Endemic in West Africa, Lassa fever is reported from Sierra Leone, Guinea, Liberia, and Nigeria. The overall case-fatality rate of Lassa fever is 1%, and the number of Lassa virus infections per year in West Africa is estimated at 100,000 to 500,000, with approximately 5,000 deaths annually (Africa CDC, 2022). The *Mastomynatalensis* species complex of rodents plays host actively to Lassa virus. Similarly, Ebola virus disease is a zoonotic disease transmitted by exposure to wildlife such as forest fruit bats. The disease manifestation is characterized by fever, bleeding, and diarrhea. Its trademark is the high morbidity and mortality rate. It was first discovered in Sub-Saharan Africa in 1976. The disease is now endemic to the region. Countries such as the DRC, Uganda, Sudan, and Gabon record regular outbreak of the disease. Like other zoonotic diseases, Ebola is a product of ecology, especially the blurring of the delineation between societies and animal habitats. The 2014 Ebola outbreak in West Africa originated in Guinea (Faleye, 2017b).

The spread of the Lassa fever and Ebola virus disease is often associated with the nature of food production and consumption in Sub-Saharan Africa. It has been observed that income and education are strong driving factors of dietary patterns in Sub-Saharan Africa (Abidoye et al., 2002). Food consumption in the African context is often associated with living standards, poverty, food security, and household resource (Obayelu et al., 2009). There are regional variations as well as rural-urban differences in food consumption patterns in Sub-Saharan Africa. The changing pattern of food consumption can be significant enough to influence the health status of any given population per time (Oyewole and Atinmo, 2015). For instance, rural dwellers in the habit of exploring the forest for varieties of bushmeat probably risk being exposed to pathogens. "Bushmeat" is a colloquial term referring to meat sourced from wild animals. It is widely consumed and traded, contributing to biodiversity loss and emergence of infectious diseases (Friant et al., 2020).

Food contamination is one of the major ways diseases are transmitted from animals to humans (Odunze et al., 2018). A rising concern for public health is the role of foods in human exposure to pathogens. Before any given food can serve as a vehicle for transmission of pathogens, it must first be contaminated by a pathogen along the food chain, from farm to fork/table. The primary sources of food contamination include irrigation water, manure, feces, soil, animals, equipment and utensils, method of harvesting, method of storage, and method of processing. In Sub-Saharan Africa, cases of food-borne illnesses are mainly focused on diagnoses to aid treatment of victims, without tracking the source of the pathogens. People are inadvertently exposed to pathogens from several sources which often cause diseases that are not reported because the symptoms are mistaken for other popular ailments such as malaria and typhoid (Mola et al., 2021; Okafor et al., 2016).

Rural-Urban Inequalities and the Management of Viral Hemorrhagic Fevers in Sub-Saharan Africa: Lessons From Lagos

The subjects of demography and public health are inherently connected. In the context of acute diseases outbreak, especially in urban areas, demographic tools could help understand epidemiological patterns. Demographic statistics reveal how social factors such as urbanization, population movements, and transition impact food security and population health. Demographic information is useful in determining required logistic support in terms of infrastructural provision and pharmaceutical distribution in line with age variances, geography, ethnicity, and socio-economic status in society (Allen and Katz, 2010). As observed by Allen and Katz (2010), public health emergency preparedness (PHEP) is based on the principle that individual health is a product of population health. Demographic analysis provides new insights into population health. Moreover, demographic information on population changes and characteristics informs public health emergency preparedness on projections of volatile geographies and vulnerable population groups. In this way, spatial demography and public health are mutually in-exclusive.

The history of the application of the demographic method to public health can be traced to the use of population statistics in public health emergency preparedness against possibilities of chemical and nuclear disasters in the United States. Urban revolution, the rapid growth of population, and landscape expansion in strategic locations of global commerce pose a major threat to population health in developing societies. As noted by Goldstein (1990: 121), "urbanization's physical and social impacts on health and disease are known . . . poor health is associated with poverty, malnutrition, poor housing, inadequate sanitation, pollution, and economic and psychological stresses, as well as with inadequate health services". It has been noted that "urban populations will continue to grow much faster than rural populations even if the urban bias in development strategies were reversed" (Hope, 1999: 47). The major impact of the urban evolution is more felt in developing countries where urbanization witnesses unprecedented vulnerabilities of the poor to industrial activities and its associated mental stress. It is argued that health promotion and the future of public health depend on the potential of public policies in addressing health issues in urban areas.

The failure of the internationalization of public health programs is evident in the partial successes recorded by WHO in terminating infectious diseases such as smallpox while other diseases persistently ravage the developing countries due to poor socio-economic and environmental conditions. This creates fertile "habitats for pathogenic microbes" (Fidler, 1997: 32). The inadequacies of national public health infrastructures in developing countries are attributable to the global and local unequal political economy of development. In the local sphere, socio-spatial disparity in resource distribution is obvious in the unequal landscape of health interventions across the rural-urban divide. Scholars have justified the lopsided investment in urban areas based on the rural-urban migration and the high density of urban population. It has been argued that the rapid population growth in cities impacts the urban environment with implications for disease processes. Unfortunately, little has been said about the political endemiology of infectious diseases such as VHFs peculiar to rural areas. For instance, the rural population is more vulnerable to zoonotic diseases due to their socio-economic activities such as food production. In the rural areas agricultural activities imply the exposure of the local population to wildlife. Across rural communities in Sub-Saharan Africa, a re-occurring reality is viral infection attributed to cultural practices rather than policy. Scholars have argued that there are existing community lifestyles that have strengthened VHFs such as Lassa fever and Ebola in the region. This includes the consumption of wildlife and poor hygiene leading to the exposure of agricultural produce to contamination by rodents (Inegbenebor et al., 2009; Wogu et al., 2019). Based on the foregoing narrative, the policy intervention engendered the tracing of exposed and infected persons as well as education on personal and environmental hygiene. These policy interventions informed by science neglect the socio-economic and political root of these re-current zoonotic disease outbreaks in Sub-Saharan Africa. Indeed, it is a colonial path dependence of the medical establishment in postcolonial Africa.

Urbanization in Africa is largely unplanned with public health consequences. The colonial era ushered in a new pattern of urban development centered on the administrative and trading cities. While colonial urbanization was unplanned at inception, the outbreaks of several infectious diseases, including the 1918–1919 influenza pandemic and the Third Plague Pandemic, led to urban planning regimes in many colonies in Africa (Swanson, 1977; Faleye, 2017a). Since the restructuring of the African landscape in colonial times, the urban areas stand at the center of power and national developmental trajectory. In examining the spatial politics of health in Sub-Saharan Africa, the control of endemic Lassa fever and EVD in Lagos, Nigeria provides a rare insight into the nature of rural-urban health inequality in the region. The population of Lagos in the colonial era rose from 99,700 in 1921 to 665,246 in 1960 (Faleye, 2017a). In the postcolonial era, based on the data of the Nigerian Population Commission, the population of Lagos rose by about 500% between 1963 and 2006 and about 700% in 2015. In 2006, the population of Lagos was 9,019,534. The estimated population of Lagos in 2021 is about 22 million. In this vein, urban land use expanded from 230.8 km² in 1976 to 805.4 km² in 2015 (Ayeni, 2016). There is a demographic shift in population distribution in Lagos over time. While the bulk of the population was located at the center of administration on the Lagos Island during the colonial period, the postcolonial era witnessed a rapid shift in population density from the center to the margins of the megacity. The case of three local governments is illustrative of this phenomenon. For instance, the population of Lagos Island and Ikeja, as centers of influence, stood at 209,437 and 313,000 respectively, whereas Alimosho, characterized by many suburban settlements, has a population of 1,277,714 (Lagos State Government, n.d.).

While the impact of the rapid growth of the population and environmental challenges affect population health in the face of the devastating pandemics and epidemics in the colonial era, the challenges of urban sprawl and poor infrastructure in the city's extension continued in the postcolonial era. However, despite the infrastructural challenges stemming from demographic changes and socio-spatial inequalities, Lagos has been able to manage public health emergencies. The nature of demographic changes in Lagos witnessed a transition of densification from the center to the periphery suburban areas. This pattern of demographic change is not commensurate with the infrastructural spread in Lagos. It showcases a pattern of socio-spatial inequalities more visible at the urban margins.

The devastating manifestation of Lassa fever disease sends jitters anytime an outbreak occurs in a metropolitan Africa of Lagos. In the face of Lassa fever virulence around Nigeria, it is common to see threatening headlines in newspapers such as "Lassa fever: What makes Lagos a bad case". In the foregoing headline of 22 February 2020, the Nigerian *Vanguard Newspaper* mirrors the state of public opinion on an LF outbreak in Lagos, thus:

> Saturday Vanguard gathered that the index case is a Law student from Eboyin state diagnosed at the Lagos University Teaching Hospital, LUTH, on February 17 and is currently in isolation at the hospital. The development was confirmed by the Lagos State Commissioner for Health Prof, Akin Abayomi. He said health authorities from the Lagos State Ministry of Health had traced 63 persons that had close contact with the index case and they were being monitored. The news sent chills down the spines of millions of Lagosians and several residents of the populous megapolis went into panic mode. Many persons have been running helterskelter in anticipation of the worst. . . . Prior to the Lagos incident, outbreaks of Lassa in Nigeria had already killed 103 people within the first seven weeks of 2020. The Nigeria Centre for Disease Control (NCDC) in its latest statistics on the virus said the overall number of confirmed cases rose by 115 last week to a total of 586 across the country. All these combined to put fear of an impending Lassa fever epidemic is palpable among the residents. Within hours of the report, the demand for hand sanitizers, household disinfectants, rat traps and rat poison in and around the city went up and the prices increased appreciably. This response was not unexpected given that it wasn't the first time that Lassa fever would hit Lagos. In several respects the disease was only making a return to the megacity.
>
> (Vanguard, 2020)

The case of population pressure in Lagos technically makes an outbreak of any infectious disease a bad case. Though Lagos has witnessed sporadic outbreaks of Lassa fever, these cases have failed to boomerang into a serious public health crisis as expected. Lagos witnessed its first case of EVD outbreak in 2014. The importer of the EVD viral disease was a Liberian national admitted to a private hospital in Lagos in July 2014. The outcome of an EVD test later proved positive. Unfortunately, the healthcare workers involved in the index case were exposed to the virus and subsequently died (Oladimeji et al., 2015). Thus, the Ebola outbreak in Lagos provides historical lessons in the context of public health preparedness in Nigeria. The history of the Ebola outbreak and control in Lagos is a history of African public health miracle. This is the case, if we put into cognizance the huge population size, of about 20 million people in the mega city of Lagos. The demographic structure of the mega city in which more than two-thirds of active youths are involved in daily hustling and bustling with very limited social distancing was enough reason to make an observer frightened at the onset of the outbreak. Moreover, public health challenges of poor healthcare delivery system and chronic problems of waste and sewerage disposal set the stage for an Ebola Armageddon in Lagos. As the US consul general to Nigeria Jeffery Hawkins puts it, "the last thing anyone in the world wants to hear is the two words 'Ebola' and 'Lagos' in the same sentence . . . that juxtaposition . . . conjured up images of an apocalyptic urban outbreak" (Boseley, 2014). The foregoing nightmare of Ebola outbreak did not materialize in Lagos.

The official responses to Lassa fever and EVD in Lagos are the product of governance. This involved the synergy between the government and the civil society in Nigeria. The official responses differ in time and the nature of outbreaks. However, these approaches converge in public health emergency responses including the contact tracing of infected persons, emergency responses to suspected cases, availability of testing centers, free provision of the treatment and the intensification of environmental sanitation exercises, and public health sensitization across the city. The Official data of the Nigerian Center for Disease Control documented the swift response of the Federal Ministry of Health in cooperation with stakeholders at the state and local government levels in Nigeria as well as international support derived from Nigerian international relations on issues of global health. In the case of Ebola, the declaration of a public health emergency redirected the attention of the health sector to resolve the public health challenges brought about by the Ebola outbreak. This declaration implies the government's commitment to allocating financial resources to curb the outbreak. The ensued contact tracing, cross-border disease surveillance, construction of new health infrastructure and renovation of existing ones to support Ebola management, as well as prompt procurement of medical supplies was a capital-intensive response.

The infrastructure provided for the polio eradication program was adapted to strengthen the public health intervention in the EVD outbreak in Lagos. This is an aspect of "accidental" public health emergency preparedness. However, the lessons of EVD led to the creation of a solid public health preparedness to tackle future EIDs (Abayomi et al., 2021). This was a timely approach by the Lagos state government in collaboration with the federal and local governments as well as international partners. This public health readiness was decisive in controlling COVID-19. As noted by Akande (2020), the first case of COVID-19 in Nigeria was a case reported in an Italian citizen who works in Nigeria and returned from Milan, Italy, to Lagos, Nigeria, on the 25th of February 2020.

In this way, the Nigerian government provided leadership in curbing the diseases. In the political context, this astute political goodwill to curb these outbreaks in Lagos was a fallout from the potent threat of the virus to all Nigerians, including the Nigerian elites, who are major investors and stakeholders in the Nigerian industrial hub and mega city – Lagos. The fear of contagion engendered benevolent local responses in support of the government's sanitary measures. This was the case of the youthful population of Lagos and the desperate vision to survive and succeed economically despite the environmental health challenges. Indeed, the cultural representation of Lagos as a refuge for all and a place of opportunity to be protected by all and at all costs is captured in the local parlance – "*Eko o nibaje*". Lassa fever and Ebola are known infectious viral hemorrhagic diseases that are spreading beyond their earlier geographical delimitations in the past 20 years. The global pattern of infectious disease morbidity is changing in line with demographic changes brought about by migration, natural growth of cities, and improved transportation technology. An important feature of these changes is the nullification of the notions of urban dichotomies. For instance, the idea of a clear line between developed and developing nations as well as the rural and the urban is blurring. This phenomenon is more visible in the cities' peripheries, which now constitute the "rural of the urban". This has implications for the spread of zoonotic diseases such as Lassa fever and Ebola, which were formerly restricted to the rural areas.

The United Nations Sustainable Development Goals – Vision 2030 emphasized a need to end poverty and other deprivations in tandem with strategies that improve health and education, reduce inequality, and spur economic growth in a way that the environment and climate are protected. Thus, rural-urban divide in health intervention unveils levels of socio-spatial inequalities and geographies of vulnerability. Bridging the rural-urban divide and associated spatial inequality in formulating public health policies is crucial for the control of viral hemorrhagic fevers in Sub-Saharan Africa.

Conclusion

This chapter shows that spatial demography, infrastructure, and governance impact public health in Sub-Saharan Africa. Here, the focus is Lagos, Nigeria's mega city with a population of about 22 million people. The impact of urbanization and demographic changes on emerging infectious diseases is more obvious in urban centers such as Lagos due to its strategic importance in the spatial demographic politics in Nigeria. The case of population pressure in Lagos technically makes an outbreak of any infectious disease a bad case. This was true in the colonial era. The question is, what changed? In the postcolonial era, though Lagos has witnessed outbreaks of viral hemor-rhagic fevers such as Lassa fever and Ebola, these cases have failed to boo-merang into a disastrous public health crisis.

The timely control of these infectious diseases' outbreaks in Lagos was a product of political good will which manifested in heavy financial invest-ment in disease control. The ability of Lagos to attract this attention is not far-fetched from its population size and geostrategic location as an important economic hub. This pattern of health intervention showcases socio-spatial inequalities more visible at the urban margins and rural areas. The Lagos miracle shows the inalienability of political goodwill in health intervention and the urgent need to bridge the rural-urban divide in public health policies in Sub-Saharan Africa.

References

Abayomi, A., Balogun, M.R., Bankole, M., Banke-Thomas, A., Mutiu, B., Olawepo, J., et al. (2021). From Ebola to COVID-19: Emergency Preparedness and Response Plans and Actions in Lagos, Nigeria. *Globalization and Health*, 17(79). https://doi.org/10.1186/s12992-021-00728-x.

Abidoye, R.O., Madueke, L.A., and Abidoye, G.O. (2002). The Relationship Between Dietary Habits and Body-Mass Index Using the Federal Airport Authority of Nige-ria as the Sample. *Nutrition and Health*, 16(3): 215–227.

Africa Center for Disease Control. (2022). Lassa Fever. https://africacdc.org/disease/lassa-fever/#:~:text=The%20overall%20case%2Dfatality%20rate,disease%20is%20not%20uniformly%20performed.

Akande, O.W. and Akande, T.M. (2020). COVID-19 Pandemic: A Global Health Burden. *National Postgraduate Medical Journal of Nigeria*, 27(3): 147–155. www.npmj.org/temp/NigerPostgradMedJ273147-50714_140514.pdf.

Allen, H. and Katz, R. (2010). Demography and Public Health Emergency Prepar-edness: Making the Connection. *Population Research and Policy Review*, 29(4): 527–539.

Asogun, D.A., Adomeh, D.I., Ehimuan, J., Odia, I., and Hass, M. (2012). Molecular Diagnostics for Lassa Fever at Irrua Specialist Teaching Hospital, Nigeria: Lessons Learnt from Two Years of Laboratory Operation. *PLoS Neglected Tropical Dis-eases*, 6(9): e1839. https://doi.org/10.1371/journal.pntd.0001839.

Ayeni, A.O. (2016). Increasing Population, Urbanization and Climatic Factors in Lagos State, Nigeria: The Nexus and Implications on Water Demand and Supply. *Journal of Global Initiatives: Policy, Pedagogy, Perspective*, 11(2). http://digital-commons.kennesaw.edu/jgi/vol11/iss2/6. Accessed 22 June 2022.

Boseley, S. (2014). Nigeria's Ebola Crackdown Is an Example to the World, 20 Octo-ber. www.theguardian.com/world/2014/oct/20/nigeria-ebola-crackdown-example-to-world. Accessed 12 November 2021.

Carter-Pokras, O., Zambrana, R.E., Mora, S.E., and Aaby, K.A. (2007). Emergency Preparedness: Knowledge and Perceptions of Latin American Immigrants. *Journal of Health Care for the Poor and Underserved*, 18(2): 465–481.

Centers for Disease Control and Prevention (CDC). (2004). Imported Lassa Fever. *Morbidity and Mortality Weekly Report*, 53(38): 894–897.

Connolly, C., Keil, R., and Ali, S.H. (2021). Extended Urbanisation and the Spatialities of Infectious Disease: Demographic Change, Infrastructure and Governance. *Urban Studies*, 58(2), 245–263.

Faleye, O.A. (2017a). Environmental Change, Sanitation and Bubonic Plague in Lagos, 1924–31. *International Review of Environmental History*, 3(2): 89–103.

Faleye, O.A. (2017b). Sociospatial Networks and Trans-Border Epidemic Surveillance in West Africa: The Ebola Outbreak of 2014–2015 in Perspective. *The Nigerian Health Journal*, 17(3): 61–69.

Faleye, O.A. (2023). COVID-19 Pandemic, Geopolitics of Health and Security Entanglement in West Africa. In Moyo, I. and Ndlovu-Gatsheri, S.J. (Eds.), *COVID-19 Pandemic and the Politics of Life*. London: Routledge.

Fidler, D.P. (1997). The Public's Health in the Global Era: Challenges, Responses, and Responsibilities. *Indiana Journal of Global Legal Studies*, 5(1): 11–51.

Foucault, M. (1982). The Subject and Power. *Critical Inquiry*, 8(4): 777–795.

Friant, S., Ayambem, W.A., Alobi, A.O., Ifebueme, N.M., Otukpa, O.M., Ogar, D.A., et al, (2020). Eating Bushmeat Improves Food Security in a Biodiversity and Infectious Disease "Hotspot". *EcoHealth*, 17(1): 125–138.

Goldstein, G. (1990). Urbanization, Health and Well-Being: A Global Perspective. *Journal of the Royal Statistical Society*, 39(2): 121–133.

Happi, A.N., Happi, C.T., and Schoepp, R.J. (2019). Lassa Fever Diagnostics: Past, Present, and Future. *Current Opinion in Virology*, 37: 132–138. https://doi.org/10.1016/j.coviro.2019.08.002.

Hope, K.P. (1999). Managing Rapid Urbanization in Africa: Some Aspects of Policy. *Journal of Third World Studies*, 16(2): 47–59.

Inegbenebor, U., Okosun, J., and Inegbenebor, J. (2009). Prevention of Lassa Fever in Nigeria. *Transactions of the Royal Society of Tropical Medicine and Hygiene*, 104: 51–54.

Lagos State Government. (n.d.). About Lagos. https://hos.lagosstate.gov.ng/about-lagos/.

Mbembe, J.A. (2003). Necropolitics. *Public Culture*, 15(1): 11–40.

Mbembe, J.A. (2019). *Necropolitics*. Durham: Duke University Press.

Mola, I., Onibokun, A., and Oranusi, S. (2021). Prevalence of Multi-drug Resistant Bacteria Associated with Foods and Drinks in Nigeria (2015–2020): A Systematic Review. *Italian Journal of Food Safety*, 10(4): 9417. https://doi.org/10.4081/ijfs.2021.9417.

Obayelu, A.E., Okoruwa, V.O., and Oni, O.A. (2009). Analysis of rural and urban households' food consumption differential in the North-Central, Nigeria: A microeconometric approach. *Journal of Development and Agricultural Economics*, 1(2): 018–026.

Odunze, E., Mikecz, O., Pica-Ciamarra, U., and Boussini, H. (2018). The Africa Sustainable Livestock 2050 Initiative. The Monetary Impact of Zoonotic Diseases on Society in Nigeria: Evidence from Four Zoonoses. Food and Agriculture Organisation. https://www.fao.org/documents/card/en/c/CA2146EN/.

Okafor, A.C., Igwesi, S.N., David, E.J., Okolo, V.K., and Agu, K. (2016). Presence of Bacteria with Pathogenic Potential among Already-Used Toothbrushes from University Students. *American Journal of Life Science Researches*, 4: 16–20.

Oladimeji, A.M., Gidado, S., Nguku, P., Nwangwu, I.G., Patil, N.D., Oladosu, and Poggensee, G. (2015). Ebola Virus Disease–Gaps in Knowledge and Practice among

Healthcare Workers in Lagos. *Tropical Medicine & International Health*, 20(9): 1162–1170.

Oyewole, O.E. and Atinmo, T. (2015). Nutrition transition and chronic diseases in Nigeria. *Proceedings of the Nutrition Society*, 74(4): 460–465.

Swanson, W.M. (1977). The Sanitation Syndrome: Bubonic Plague and Urban Native Policy in the Cape Colony, 1900–1909. *Journal of African History*, 18, (3): 387–410.

Vanguard. (2020). Lassa Fever: What Makes Lagos a Bad Case, 22 February. www. vanguardngr.com/2020/02/lassa-fever-what-makes-lagos-a-bad-case/. Accessed 24 June 2021.

Walker, D.H., Mccormick, J.B., Johnson, K.M., Webb, P.A., Komba-Kono, G., Elliott, L.H., and Gardner, J.J. (1982). Pathologic and Virologic Study of Fatal Lassa Fever in Man. *American Journal of Pathologists*, 107: 349–356.

Wogu, J.O., Chukwu, C.O., Nwafor, K.A., et al. (2019). Mass Media Reportage of Lassa Fever in Nigeria: A Viewpoint. *Journal of International Medical Research*, 48: 1–7.

Part II

Church Administration and the Religious Determinants of Health

5 Socio-Economic Dynamics of Covid-19 Pandemic, Church Administration, and Social Welfare in Nigeria

Peter O. Alokan and Opeyemi Aluko

Introduction

A significant number of pandemics and epidemics have been recorded in human history. The most recent of these pandemics is Covid-19, which was first discovered in China and reported by the World Health Organization (WHO) in November 2019. Like other pandemics, Covid-19 has had enormous negative impacts on the health, economy, education, political structure, and security in West Africa (Faleye, 2023). Not only did the Covid-19 pandemic lead to concurrent lockdown experiences that captured many nations, it also had a significant impact on religion and religious practices in different nations. Also, the crisis has generated different speculations and controversies in different quarters of the world.

The Christ Apostolic Church, as a faith-based institution, has responded to pandemics and epidemics in different ways throughout the history of the world. For instance, when the Black Death struck Europe in 1347, it crumbled feudalism. The church struggled to cope with the plague's damaging consequences and its reputation suffered as a result (Thompson, 2008). These developments stimulated secularism and the birth of the modern international system.

Moreover, in the Protestant Reformation era, when the plague struck in Europe, the church responded differently. In Wittenberg, Martin Luther responded that prayers of faith should be offered up for God's mercy along with responsible practices of sanitation, medication, self-quarantine, and social distancing to help stop the spread. Notwithstanding the effects of the plagues on the church, Christians like Luther did not close their doors to anyone who needed care at the time. Similarly, during the 1918 Spanish Flu, church buildings in affected areas of the USA were closed while believers continued worshipping from house to house. Some churches opened their doors to serve as health clinics as hospitals were bursting with increase in affected patients. Many Christians sacrificed their lives to provide care for the sick (Whiting, 2020).

The Christ Apostolic Church since its emergence in Nigeria has witnessed some pandemics and epidemics and the church has responded to the events

DOI: 10.4324/9781003429135-8

of the pandemics in different ways. Before Covid-19, the CAC witnessed the 1918 Influenza and 2014 Ebola virus especially within the Nigerian context. In 1918, the Christ Apostolic Church was still a Prayer Group (*Egbe Aladura*). Historians of the emergence of the Aladura Pentecostal Movement affirmed that the religious practices of faith for divine healing, fervent prayers, and obedience to prophetic injunctions offered by new rising Aladura prophets in Southwest Nigeria were instrumental to the testimony and miracles of the affected patients of the 1918 influenza epidemic (Ademakinwa, 2012). There is no doubt, Sophia Odulami played a significant role in bringing people to Christ without the use of orthodox medicine or herbs and charms. Sophia Odulami received a divine revelation with the use of rain water for healing. Ademakinwa (2012) confirmed that many people in Southwest Nigeria, especially in Isoyin and Ijebu-Ode, who used the rain water for diverse ailments got cured.

This trend of development placed the Prayer Group darlings of the people since they enjoyed healing without any cost implication. While the colonial administrators were closing down schools, hospitals, clinic, offices, as well as some churches and a good number of missionaries were abandoning their congregation to heed the call to go back home (Ayegboyin and Ishola, 1997), it was the Prayer Group that rose up to the task of delivering the people from death through their prayers and faith in divine healing. The belief of this new Aladura Group is that God is capable of healing any form of sickness if his people would only trust in him solely. This theological idea has become well developed in the doctrines and tenets of the Aladura Pentecostal church, especially the Christ Apostolic Church. In fact, divine healing is at the hub of the religious practice of the church all through its existence. Remarkably, this religious practice brought the church to further limelight in the 1930s especially through the 1930 Aladura Pentecostal revivals which erupted at Oke-Ooye, Ilesa, Southwest Nigeria.

During the Ebola epidemic in Nigeria, the Christ Apostolic Church, like other Aladura churches, continued in the belief in divine healing through the prayer of faith. The use of water especially for washing of hand as recommended by the Ministry of Health in Nigeria synchronizes in some way with the Aladura, who already believe in the potency of water as a healing agent. While the church encouraged adherence to the hand-washing rules of the Ministry of Health, the congregants were instructed to the discipline and practice of vigorous prayers and belief in God as the only divine healer. It is believed that the Aladura prayer mode is a shield against diverse forms of diseases, including the Ebola virus. This chapter examines the disruptions of Covid-19 in Nigeria and local responses, especially in church administration and social welfare with reference to Christ Apostolic Church.

Poverty Cycle and Covid-19 Gauge in Nigeria

The classical view of poverty was perceived by Adam Smith (1776). He purported that poverty is the inability of someone to possess the required resources to purchase some necessities required by nature or custom. This view is a generalized overview that has encapsulated the entire world to be poor because nobody is self-sufficient by nature and might not be able to get a basic necessity at a particular time though he has the wherewithal. Poverty, as opined by Sen (1981), is the absolute deprivation in terms of a person's capabilities to get basic necessities of life which emanates from relative deprivation in terms of commodities, incomes, policies, and resources. This view implies that relative deprivation is a process of incurring poverty that proceeds to absolute deprivation. This assertion corroborates what Peter Townsend defines poverty to be. He said it is what starts as a purely relative measure of deprivation or lack of the resources necessary to facilitate the participation of an individual in the activities, customs, and food commonly approved by the community (Townsend, 1979).

Other contemporary scholars such as Bluemenstock (2016) view poverty as a relative phenomenon, where someone's resources are so negligible and seriously below the requirement for survival for the average individual or family that they are excluded from the regular mode of living and association, customs and activities. This view strongly emphasized social exclusion as a fundamental yardstick for poverty. Resources availability is stressed, especially when they are seriously below average as a symptom of relative poverty. The World Bank 'standard method' used to measure poverty is based on incomes or the consumption levels of individuals or households. Therefore, a person is considered poor if his or her consumption or income level falls below a certain minimum level and which incapacitate in meeting basic needs such as daily balanced meal, good clothing, adequate transportations, good housing, portable drinking water, good health, and educational facilities. When estimating poverty worldwide, the same benchmark poverty line has to be used and expressed in a common unit across countries. Therefore, for the purpose of global aggregation and comparison, the World Bank uses the yardstick set between $1.25 and $2 per day. This implies that any person living below the minimum level, which is usually called the poverty line, is poor. However, this measurement might not be pronounced in the developed countries like United Kingdom (UK) and United States of America (USA) among others as compared to the developing countries of Africa and other parts of the world.

The perspective of the European Commission (2021) on poverty is that people are judged to be poor if their income and resources are very inadequate or insufficient. Due to the poverty level, they are susceptible to experiencing multiple disadvantages through unemployment, low income, poor housing, inadequate healthcare, and barriers to lifelong learning, culture, sport, and recreation. This perception of poverty might essentially be applicable to European nations, but a more comprehensive and balanced view of poverty encompasses all regions of the world. It opines that poverty includes lack of income and productive resources to ensure sustainable livelihoods, hunger and malnutrition, ill health, limited or lack of access to education and other basic services, increased morbidity and mortality from illness, homelessness and inadequate housing, and unsafe environments and social discrimination and exclusion; it is also characterized by lack of participation in decision making and in civil, social and cultural life (United Nations, n.d.).

Poverty reveals the level of misery in a country. The misery index is the sum of the unemployment rate, the lending rate, and the inflation rate minus the percent change in real GDP per capita of a country (Szmigiera, 2021). Among the countries ranked in his 2018 edition, Nigeria, South Africa, and Egypt are in the top 10 of most miserable countries. Nigeria, for instance, has one of Africa's highest unemployment rates with 23% of its population, that is, 18 million of the labour force, currently without jobs. The inflation rate in Nigeria and in Egypt are 11% and 14%, respectively (Anoba, 2019). In 2020, Nigeria overtook India as the country with the highest number of people living in extreme poverty. Covid-19 pandemic effect has a global reckoning (Ciotti et al., 2020). Covid-19 had increased the level of poverty in many countries including Nigeria (Boettke and Powell, 2021).

The period of lockdown further impacted on the already weak forces of demand and supply in the open market to be shut down and others operate far below average. Inflation level increased from an unbearable level to a more volatile level, where food availability and affordability level of households become depleted. The gross weakness and inefficient and poor infrastructure of the health sector was exposed. Before the advent of Covid-19, the upper class and government officials in the country do neglect the national health infrastructure for medical tourism abroad; however, they are forced to face the adverse effect of the lacuna caused by the extent of neglect of the dilapidated health facility. Covid-19 as well exposed the weakness of the government in responding to human need at the time of distress. Covid-19 therefore made poverty to become more entrenched in the country and keeps roving in a cycle. The subsequent sections examine the role of non-state actors in mitigating the socio-economic and medical challenges posed by Covid-19 in Nigeria. The focus is Christ Apostolic Church and its Covid-19 intervention.

Covid-19 Disruptions: The Nigerian Experience

Nigeria recorded her first index case of Covid-19 on 27 February 2020 when an Italian citizen visiting Lagos tested positive for the virus. On 9 March 2020 a second case of the virus was confirmed in Ewekoro Ogun State. This time it was a Nigerian citizen who had contact with the Italian citizen. Since then, the nation has experienced four major waves of the spread of the coronavirus. Within the first two months of the first wave, Nigeria had recorded 3,912 confirmed cases, with 679 recoveries and 117 deaths. From February 27 to December 15, when the second wave was already announced, there were 74,132 recorded Covid-19 cases. Among this, 66,494 recovered, while 1,200 lives were lost to the crisis (Worldometer, 2021). The third and fourth waves of the viral spread witnessed a rise in the disease morbidity and fatality in Nigeria (The Guardian, 21 December 2021).

Nigeria recorded series of lockdowns during the first wave. The first ever reported lockdown experience associated with the pandemic began effectively on the midnight of Monday 30 March 2020. This first phase lasted for two weeks. The lockdown affected Lagos, Ogun, and Abuja majorly. During these weeks, all major institutions in these states were completely shut down with the essential service providers like the media houses, police stations, and petrol stations, among others, left to continue to function. The citizens were mandated to stay at home. A social distance rule, use of face mask, washing of hands with soap and water in a prescribed manner, and use of hand sanitizers were among other measures raised by the Ministry of Health in Nigeria and the Task Force set up by the federal government as well as each state government to prevent the spread of the virus.

The Nigerian experience was quite severe at the initial stage of the prevention program for the spread of the virus and the lockdown experience, that is, from April through May 2020. The reason for this according to some observers is the poor state of the masses even before the outbreak of the virus (Garba, 2020). Another factor mentioned concurrently is the weak state of institutions that should help in curbing the spread, especially the hospitals at all levels. There was also lack of adequate social welfare programs that should cater for the needs of the poor majority. This should have constrained them to observe the stipulations raised by the government, especially the observance of the total lockdown. The citizens became vulnerable and more people were affected. For fear of financial and economic collapse, people began to buy and hoard household utilities, essential food, and commodity items.

The total lockdown closed down many businesses. Some business owners asked their employees to work from home to reduce operation costs. Some privately owned institutions cut down the size of their staff, while some cut down the wages of their employees. As the days of lockdown increased, private school owners could no longer pay their teachers and other staff, among other challenges (Faleye, 2023). The suffering was no longer about survival from Covid-19 but how to sustain family finances. The Covid-19 pandemic also affected the social life of the masses in Nigeria. Entertainment centers were practically shut down. All sporting activities were stopped. All social events and gatherings were practically given away to the extent that those who attempted any form of gathering were sanctioned and penalized by the government. There was also a threat to the security of the nation as bandits, militia groups, cultists and hoodlums used the opportunity to cause havoc in some states. (Faleye, 2023).

Apart from the economic and social effects of the Nigerian Covid-19 experience, the religious life of the masses was also threatened. The pandemic led to a complete shutdown of all places of worship, including churches, mosques, and even African Traditional worship centers. Owing to the fact that Nigerians are very religious and are not used to virtual worship, many worshipers found it difficult to cope with Covid-19 regulations of physical distancing and gathering of not more than 20 people. It must be noted that Nigerians always appear physically during their religious meetings and this has been one of the ways of revealing their religiosity, this aspect of the experience affected the masses more. Religion has been one of the ways the masses survive through times of economic hardship, grief, pain, and the like.

Notably, the second wave of the coronavirus crisis in Nigeria was announced a little while after the masses began to get a sigh of relief after the lockdown experience was eased by the Government. In the Covid-19 Presidential Task Force briefing held on 12 September 2020, Dr. Osagie Ehanire, the Nigerian Minister of Health mentioned that Nigeria cannot afford to rejoice or speak of success as a result dwindling figures of the positive cases of the Covid-19. He noted that countries that were reported to have defeated Covid-19 were at the time experiencing an upsurge in cases of the spread of the virus. This new experience was identified as the second wave (Efem, 2021). To this end, the Minister advised citizens to continue to adhere to the Covid-19 protocols and other health-related instruction to avoid a second wave of infections. Notwithstanding this admonition, towards the end of 2020, the Media announced that Nigeria entered a second wave of Coronavirus infection. The news came when Boss Mustapha, the secretary to the Government of Nigeria and the Chairman of the Covid-19 Presidential Task Force raised the alarm in a briefing (Berker, 2020). At the time of his briefing, more than 76,000 cases have been diagnosed with the virus and 1,201 victims have been reported dead.

Although, Nigeria did not fall back to another stage of lockdown, still the news of the second wave affected lots of businesses as many business owners and enterprises became very meticulous in their approach to work. Government offices were also affected as public servants below grade level 12 were advised to work from their homes (BBC, 2021). Public and private primary and secondary schools that were opened recently were asked to close for the session earlier than expected. Although it was not announced publicly, Nigeria has been experiencing economic recession since this very time. The second wave also affected the social life of the citizen remarkably. People were asked to avoid social gatherings, like it was in the first wave. The second wave had serious impacts on Christian worshipers because it came towards the end of the year and it also affected the preparation towards Christmas, the New Year holidays, and festivities. For instance, the 2020 Christmas and Boxing Day celebrations were held in a low–key manner in different parts of the nation. Religious worship was also affected as churches and mosques were asked to adhere to the Covid-19 protocols instituted for churches and mosques earlier. In Lagos state, the experience left a mark on religious worship on 31 December 2020 because religious institutions could not observe the usual Crossover night service into the New Year 2021. The Crossover service has been the tradition of churches in Nigeria. After a long debate with the government, churches were only permitted to observe a service in the evening keeping all the Covid-19 protocols.

Covid-19 Disruptions and the Christ Apostolic Church

In line with the constitution of Christ Apostolic Church, Nigeria (CAC), CAC is an Independent Pentecostal Church whose birth is traceable to the indigenous Pentecostal brand that emerged in Ijebu-Ode, Southwest of Nigeria, called the Prayer Band (*Egbe Aladura*) in 1918 (Alokan, 2011). Technically, Aladura is a classification of churches that holds an indigenous African type of Pentecostal Christianity similar to but not the same as the Pentecostalism that emerged in the Azusa Street Revival on 9 April 1906 in Los Angeles, led by William Seymour, an African American preacher (Poloma, 1982). It has been noted that the Aladura began as a prophetic movement. Different prophetic figures contributed to the emergence of the early Aladura. They include Joseph Shadare, the leader of the 1918 Prayer Band (*Egbe Aladura*) and the Precious Stone Society, Sophia Odunlami Ajayi of the Precious Stone Society, Joseph Ayo Babalola and Daniel Orekoya, who were the major agents of the 1930 Aladura Pentecostal revivals, among others (Ayegboyin and Ishola, 1997). Undoubtedly, the 1930 revivals were a major landmark in the Aladura Pentecostal history. This revival aided the rapid spread of the Aladura Pentecostal Faith, especially the religious practice of prayer and divine healing, throughout Nigeria and many parts of Africa. The Aladura Pentecostal revival movement grew to become the Christ Apostolic Church in 1943. Owing to this, the Christ Apostolic Church could be regarded not only as an Aladura Pentecostal Church but are of the first Aladura churches in Nigeria because its origin is directly linked to the 1918 Prayer Revivals of the *Egbe Aladura* (Prayer Band) of 1918 (Alokan et al., 2011). The root of the Christ Apostolic Church in the Egbe Aladura prayer band is of vital importance as the year 1918 marked the outbreaks of the Influenza pandemic – a major public health emergency that stimulated prayer revivals around the world.

In Nigeria, authorities implemented public health regulations to control the pandemic. The church's responses to this public health regulation provide a vital ground to measure the impact of these regulations. Like all other religious institutions in Nigeria, CAC bore the brunt of the Covid-19 pandemic in different ways. In an online Focus Group Discussion (FGD) carried out among members of the Christ Apostolic Church Oke-Iyanu, Odemuyiwa District, Lagos, and Christ Apostolic Church, Source of Blessing, Idimu Camp District, Lagos,[1] on the possible outcomes of the lockdown, especially when it would be eased down finally by the government, it was observed that the closure of different local assemblies from April to July led to loss of zeal for congregational worship among members. It also led to the migration of members to other churches. The FGD also revealed that the lockdown has already created a gap in the pastor-church member relationships that existed before and limited the pastoral care offered to members especially those that live far away from the church environment.

Although the lockdown of the churches was the primary consequence of the ordeal, this came with different issues on church administration and the responsibility of the church to the congregants and the society, especially as it pertains to social welfare. Despite the close of public and physical worship which made the online church meetings more relevant, it was obvious that the e-worship cannot replace or substitute for physical worship in different CAC assemblies. Before the lockdown, the pandemic led to a drastic reduction in the time allotted for church meetings, thus a disruption to church worship. Most of the church meetings scheduled for two to three hours had to be trimmed to 30 minutes or one hour at most. Churches that hold more than a service on Sunday had to limit their worship to a single, one-hour online meetings. Church conferences and conventions that were scheduled to be held during the lockdown were shelved, while some programs were held virtually.

While the online meetings were not really new to many Charismatic churches in Lagos and Abeokuta, the case was different for most CAC assemblies. For instance, many Christ Apostolic Church assemblies even those in the cities had to start learning how to run an online church meeting during the lockdown period. Holding an online meeting was not only the issue, getting members to participate was also very difficult. This is because going by the CAC tradition in Nigeria, the church has been primarily designed for physical meetings purposely to meet the needs of the grassroots. The online meetings were not only new but according to members of Christ Apostolic Church, Odemuyiwa District, Lagos, they do not look real.[2] One major factor that estranged the use of the new model was the number of adults in the church who were not social media inclined. The old generation of Christ Apostolic Church, which constitutes almost 50% of the church, considers social media as a tool that promotes social vices. Only the younger generation sees this otherwise. Since the church is practically managed and led by the older generation, it was difficult for most of the local assemblies to switch to online services easily. Only local assemblies led by ministers from the younger generation were able to transition from the traditional method of worship to the new model. However, this religious position was reconsidered by many CAC faithful during the latter part of the lockdown.

Likewise, CAC is a revival meeting-driven church. The kinds of services held were not restricted to Sunday services alone. Weeklong revival meetings, vigils, large group crusades, and prayer retreats on Prayer Mountains were often conducted. All of these were completely stopped. Although some ministers tried to host revival meetings using online platforms, especially when the government still permitted gatherings of not less than 20 people, the result was not in any way compared to what was the norm before the Covid-19 experience. Christ Apostolic Church leadership also suspended different large group meetings. All CAC seminaries in Nigeria were shut down; the Pastor Training and Ordination program, revival meetings on Prayer Mountains, CAC Annual Camp Meeting and other programs were suspended. These disruptions created a huge burden for the CAC administrators. Indeed, the experience was unprecedented in the history of the church. Another side to the experience as it pertains to CAC is the financial challenge that came with the experience. Unlike some Charismatic churches where collection of church offerings was through online transfer and the likes, the CAC is used to collect offerings physically. Consequently, the CAC faced the challenge of low and reduced income and high church expenditure. This experience was not only limited to the CAC but virtually all of Aladura Pentecostal, which has the highest number of low-class and middle-class Nigerian citizens; coupled with the different economic challenges they could not surmount at the time, tithe and offerings reduced drastically.

Not only did most church pastors have to cater for the needs of members who became helpless at the time, they also had to make sure that the church facilities continue to function during the lockdown period to avoid a complete collapse. Within their household, they also encountered the challenge of meeting their needs because there was no means to get their salaries paid. Most Aladura pastors, especially the full-time ministers, could not meet up with the needs of their families. They had to rely on the benevolence of their well-to-do members. Indeed, the Covid-19 crisis has raised different questions on the full-time ministries, which do not permit the pastors to engage in other ventures that could cushion their financial base as is the case of other Pentecostal church ministers. It is obvious that the bi-vocational ministers have sources of income than the full-time ministers and can survive without much support from the church.[3] This serves as a lesson to the full-time ministers to buckle up and not rely only on the church for survival. Of course, Covid-19 economic challenges and the diversification into other means of livelihood reduce ministerial commitment to spirituality and church activities.

There is no doubt that Covid-19 with all its disruptions gave CAC the chance to review different policies and practices of the church. In the area of social welfare, Covid-19 helped the church to identify the needy among the congregation; it also helped different assemblies to reach out to the needy in their society at different levels. Although at the initial stage of the lockdown, some churches were unable to fulfil their responsibility to the congregants and the society, several church assemblies introduced different forms of social welfare programs to reduce the plight of the masses in the society. For instance, Rachel Oyeniran and Adebiyi Seye, ministers of Christ Apostolic Church, Miracle Centre, Love of God Zone, Lagos, described how the church raised funds for the needy, widows, and other members of their local assemblies in the face of the lockdown.[4] Likewise, Adejare Olorunsuyi of CAC Oke-Iyanu, Odemuyiwa District, reiterated how the church gave welfare packages to different needy families in the church as well as the youth in their community.[5] In this way, the Christ Apostolic Church served as an agency of public health by alleviating poverty and cushioning the effect of the public health regulations on the local society.

Administrative Responses of CAC to the Covid-19 Experience

Recourse to prayer for divine healing and protection against viral infection continued in CAC until the eruption of the Covid-19 pandemic in Nigeria and the world at large. However, at this time, especially due to the extent of the lockdown procedure enacted by the Nigerian government, the immediate response of the Christ Apostolic Church to the Covid-19 crisis from late March and early April was that of respect and obedience to law. CAC leadership issued a circular that mandated all local assemblies to follow to the letter all the instructions of the government and the Covid-19 Task Force. Even while some churches in different parts of Nigeria were still holding their Sunday services, the CAC local assemblies were closed as a way of supporting the effort of the government towards curbing the spread of the virus. Later, other circulars were issued at different regions of the church based on the regulations of the Task Force on the peculiarities of each state of the nation. Likewise, when the lockdown was eventually relaxed and church was opened again in late August 2020, the CAC authorities made sure each local assembly adhered to the official rules released by the government.

Another way the Christ Apostolic Church responded to the Covid-19 lockdown experience was by creating new models for church services and meetings. Some of the existing workable models were also modeled to fit into the current trend. While the church was waiting for the nation's return to normalcy, different aspects of the church life that were already functional were intensified. This includes House Fellowship Meetings and Family Prayer Altars. The use of the *Living Water* (CAC devotional resource material) was intensified. This material became the tool for collective worship in homes and cell meetings designed by some local assemblies. The CAC Sunday School Pamphlet also became a tool for Christian guidance in the cell fellowship.

The new models that were created centered on the use of online platforms. Although this came later in the period of the lockdown, different local assemblies created new online group platforms through WhatsApp, Facebook, Telegram, and Free Conference Call platforms, among others. Church meetings, especially Bible studies and prayer meetings, were held using these platforms. Some ministers of the church aired pre-recorded messages online, especially using the Facebook live platform. Apart from this, the Christ Apostolic Church was able to achieve all her slated programs for the year, especially the annual conferences. Virtual conferences were held at the CAC Headquarters' Chapel, and a reasonable amount of the online-savvy members were engaged online. Most remarkable is the effort of the CAC General Evangelist who created an online network that reached out to the world through the different revival programs hosted by the CAC. Indeed, through this platform the media team of Prophet Oladare Hezekiah, alongside the CAC Media Department, was able to capture lots of CAC members in Nigeria and abroad. This agency fostered the continuity of the revival spirit the church exemplified within the religious community in Nigeria. This also stimulated many ministers towards creating better online content for their followers.

The CAC also intensified her religious practice of prayers for divine healing. The Aladura Pentecostal concept of divine healing dates back to the early Aladura revivals in 1918. It is believed that healing could be received divinely through faith without recourse to any form of medicine for whatever diseases or ailments. The concept was first tested and proven during the 1918 Influenza in Ijebu-Ode and other parts of Southwest Nigeria. Church historians assert that the Aladura were able to provide needed healing for those who were infected, and this was done without the use of orthodox and tradition medicines (Ademakinwa, 2012). The same happened during the 1930 revivals. Based on the past outcomes, the Aladura set a model for divine healing without the use of orthodox or traditional (herbal) medicines. To this end, revivals of prayers were held online for the nation and for the healing of infected patients of Covid-19, especially those in the hospitals and isolation centers. The church prayed to curb the spread of the virus. During the lockdown, as a measure of pastoral care, some ministers asked their members to come to the church on Sunday in batches primarily to be prayed for. Pastors also visited the homes of their members to pray for them. After the lockdown was eased and members returned to their various local assemblies, keen attention was also given to prayers to curb the spread of the virus.

Remarkably, in the online Focus Group Discussion, carried out among the members of Christ Apostolic Church, the religious practice of prayer topped the list among the factors that helped the contributors to go through the tensions that came with the spread of the Covid-19 as well as the economic hardship that ensued. While 60% of the 25 contributors to the online survey carried out on who is responsible for curbing the Covid-19 crisis in Nigeria suggest that the church is responsible, 30% opine that it is the responsibility of the government and 10% hold that it is the joint responsibility of the church. Most of the contributors in the first group comment that the church has lost its power and potency as an agent for divine healing. Particular reference was made to the role the church played during the 1918 Influenza. Unarguably, the Covid-19 experience in Nigeria made many religious people to shift their focus from the church as a religious institution, especially as it regards getting healed through stipulated religious practices as means of protection from the virus and cure when infected, to building their faith on God directly. They believe instead of waiting on the government (and the church) to provide solution to the problems, people should rather look unto God. This provided a psychological succor in the early period of the pandemic when biomedicine did not understand the pathology of the disease.

Conclusion

The Covid-19 pandemic and religion is still a very recent discussion in the literature. This chapter evaluates the impact of public health measures deployed to contain the outbreak in Nigeria. It also reflects on the place of the church as an agency of public health in local communities. The focus is the Christ Apostolic Church in Nigeria. The study reveals that the pandemic and health interventions impacted church attendance, spiritual growth, administrative standard, and the social welfare of members in Nigeria. However, the economic challenge gradually fades off in line with the relaxation of public health measures. Indeed, there has been a certain level of compliance with the public health protocols, especially after the return to church worship in different assemblies in August 2020. This chapter unveils the relationship of the state and the church in a time of pandemic. This is true in strengthening their partnership on the mediums of educating the masses on disease prevention and control. The pandemic has raised the crucial issue of the need for changes in different religious positions and practices in 21st-century Nigeria.

Notes

1 Online Focus Group Discussion (FGD), WhatsApp (Social Media Application). www.whatsapp.com/cac-oke-iyanu-odemuyiwa, www.whatsapp.com/the-blacksmith-house. 6 June 2020 to 20 June 2020. A total number of 20 people participated in the FGD. The FGD was also carried out through direct call by the researcher. Five ministers participated in this category.
2 Interactions with members of the church like Deaconess Mogbojuri, Elder Thomas Ojenike, Pastor Olorunsuyi Adejare, and Tosin Akinyele, among others, from May to June 2020. This local assembly held online WhatsApp Sunday service and prayer meetings. The pastor and leaders of the meetings sent audio and text notes to members on the platform.
3 Online FGD carried out on the social media application, WhatsApp. www.whatapp.com/cac-oke-iyanu-odemuyiwa, www.whatsapp.com/the-blacksmith-house. 6 June 2020 to 20 June 2020.
4 Adebiyi Seye and Rachel Oyeniran. Interview on the Lockdown Experience of the CAC. *CAC Theological Seminary*. Lagos Campus, 15 October 2020.
5 Adejare Olorunsuyi. Interview on the Lockdown Experience of CAC, Oke-Iyanu, Odemuyiwa District, Akinyele Region, Lagos. CAC Oke-Iyanu, Lagos, 4 November 2020.

References

Ademakinwa, J.A. (2012). *History of the Christ Apostolic Church: The Faith of Our Fathers*. Grand Prairie: International Missions.

Alokan, A.J. (2011). *Christ Apostolic Church @ 90*. Ile-Ife: Timade Venture.

Alokan, P.O., Alabi, A.O., and Babalola, S.F. (2011). Critical Analyses of Church Politics and Crises Within the Indigenous Christianity in Nigeria. *American Journal of Social and Management Sciences*, 2(4): 360–370.

Anoba, I.B. (2019). Misery Index Ranks Nigeria and South-Africa as Africa's Most Miserable Countries. https://www.africanliberty.org/2019/04/11/misery-index-ranks-nigeria-and-south-africa-as-africas-most-miserable-countries/.

Ayegboyin, D. and Ishola, A. (1997). *African Indigenous Churches: An Historical Perspective*. Lagos: Greater Heights Publications.

BBC News. (2021). Coronavirus in Nigeria: Goment Guidelines for Workers, Office and Business to Check Second Wave of Coronavirus, 4 January 2021. Accessed 7 February 2021.

Berker, M. (2020). Nigeria Hit by Second Wave of Covid-19. *Anadolu Agency*, 18 December 2020. Accessed 7 February 2021.

Bluemenstock, J.E. (2016). Fighting Poverty with Data. *Science*, 353(6301): 753–754.

Boettke, P. and Powell, B. (2021). The Political Economy of the COVID-19 Pandemic. *Southern Economic Journal*, 87(4): 1090–1106.

Ciotti, M., Ciccozzi, M., Terrinoni, A., Jiang, W.C., Wang, C.B., and Bernardini, S. (2020). The COVID-19 Pandemic. *Critical Reviews in Clinical Laboratory Sciences*, 57(6), 365–388.

Efem, B. (2021). Minister of Health Admonishes Nigerians to Continue to Adhere to Covid-19 Protocols and Health Advisories to Avoid Second Wave of Infections. *Federal Ministry of Health*. Accessed 7 February 2021.

European Commission. (2021). Joint Report by the Commission and the Council on Social Inclusion. https://data.consilium.europa.eu/doc/document/ST-7301-2021-INIT/en/pdf.

Faleye, O.A. (2023). COVID-19 Pandemic, Geopolitics of Health and Security Entanglement in West Africa. In Moyo, I. and Ndlovu-Gatsheri, S.J. (Eds.), *COVID-19 Pandemic and the Politics of Life*. London: Routledge.

Garba, H.M. (2020). Covid-19 and the Challenge of False Information. *Post Covid-19 Survival (Virtual) Seminar ECWA Theological Seminary, Igbaja and CBC Africa, Zoom (An Online Platform)*, 22–24 September.

The Guardian. (2021). Nigeria Now in Fourth Wave of COVID-19 Says NCDC, 21 December. https://guardian.ng/news/nigeria-now-in-fourth-wave-of-covid-19-says-ncdc/. Accessed 23 August 2022.

Poloma, M. (1982). *The Charismatic Movement: Is There a New Pentecost?* Woodbridge: Twayne Publishers.

Sen, A. (1981). *Poverty and Famines: An Essay on Entitlement and Deprivation*. Oxford: Oxford University Press.

Smith, A. (1776). *An Inquiry into the Nature and Causes of the Wealth of Nations*. Indianapolis: Liberty Classics.

Szmigiera, M. (2021). Most Miserable Countries in the World 2020. https://www.statista.com/statistics/227162/most-miserable-countries-in-the-world/.

Thompson, L. (2008). Black Death. In Ackermann, M.E., Upshur, J.-H.L., Schroeder, M.J., Whitters, M.F., and Terry, J.J. (Eds.), *Encyclopedia of World History*. New York: Infobase Publishing.

Townsend, P. (1979). *Poverty in the United Kingdom: A Survey of Household Resources and Standards of Living*. London: Penguin.

United Nations. (n.d.). Poverty Eradication. https://www.un.org/development/desa/socialperspectiveondevelopment/issues/poverty-eradication.html#:~:text=Poverty%20entails%20more%20than%20the,of%20participation%20in%20decision%2Dmaking.

Whiting, M. (2020). Pandemics and the Church: What Does History Teach Us? Campus News, Dallas Baptist University. https://www.dbu.edu/news/2020/03/pandemics-and-the-church-what-does-history-teach-us.html.

Worldometer. (2021). Coronavirus Updates. Accessed 16 December 2020 and 7 February 2021.

6 Social Determinants of Health

The Contributions of the Catholic Church to Healthcare Delivery in Postcolonial Nigeria

Josephine Balogun and Emmanuel Okla

Introduction

The Catholic Church has constantly provided countries in West Africa and Nigeria in particular with formalised healthcare services since 1895, when the first standard hospital was built in Lantoro, Egbaland of Abeokuta, by a Catholic male Religious Congregation, SMA (SMA – Société des Missions Africaines – Society of African Missions). They were French missionaries. The hospital presently bears the name Sacred Heart Catholic Hospital, Abeokuta. The Commitment of the Catholic Church in Nigeria continued till the postcolonial era. As the British colony expanded their administration, it needed English speakers since its business associates spoke English. Therefore, Irish fathers increased in 1905 (Wall, 2018). According to the report of the health unit of the Catholic Secretariat of Nigeria in 2020, there were already over 440 Catholic healthcare facilities, ranging from clinics, primary health centres to hospitals spread across the nooks and crannies of the country, including the rural, urban slum settlements and riverine communities and the hard-to-reach areas. The Roman Catholic Church dominated other religious missions that provided a healthcare delivery system, accounting for about 40% of the total number of mission-based hospitals in 1960. At that time also, the mission healthcare facilities outnumbered those of the government. The mission hospitals were 118, while the government hospitals were 101. In about 1954, almost all the hospitals in the mid-western part of Nigeria were controlled by the Roman Catholic missions (The Library of Congress of Country Studies and CIA World Fact Book, 1991).

The Catholic Church took her initiative in practical charity in caring for the sick and building health facilities, taking the cue from Jesus Christ, whom she holds as her founder. Jesus gave his followers authority over unclean spirits with the power to drive them out and cure all kinds of diseases and illnesses. Again, he charged them to cure the sick, raise the dead, cleanse those suffering virulent-skin diseases, and drive out devils (Matthew 10:1, 8a). The notion of human dignity is at the heart of Catholic Social Teaching (CST). Immanuel Kent, a philosopher, puts human dignity by saying that while we can treat objects and animals as means to serve our needs, we should not

DOI: 10.4324/9781003429135-9

treat human beings as ends in themselves and never only as a means (Kant, 1996). The Catholic Church always has, everywhere she engages in her work of evangelisation, carried along the mission of spreading the Gospel with the social dimension of the human person, the educational, health, justice and peace development of human society.

Nigeria as a country gained independence on 1 October 1960. At that point, some health facilities were already built by the Catholic Church across the country. These facilities welcomed and still welcome all people who visit them, irrespective of their religious beliefs, race or tribes. However, the very poor ones who cannot afford the payment of their treatment are allowed to go home without pay, and sometimes they are given either money or food items to sustain them in their covalent state. Catholic missionaries, who were already working in the health institutions across the countries, got financial help to sustain their work in Nigeria. Some got support from their home countries in the form of drugs, medical equipment and even helping to train the Nigerians who were working in such healthcare systems. This offered some of the workers the opportunity to travel abroad for quality training with full scholarship. After the trainings, they returned to impact positively on the country's healthcare system through the Catholic healthcare system.

Barely seven years since Nigeria gained independence from the British government in 1967, the country witnessed a civil war that required, more than ever, the services of Nigeria's health personnel and health facilities. The civil war was attributed to the political, ethnic and religious differences in which Southeastern Nigeria wanted to secede to form the Republic of Biafra. During the war, Catholic mission hospitals provided medical care and missionaries, mainly Catholic reverend sisters, worked to treat violence survivors. The sisters, who were surgeons, physicians, nurses and midwives, as well as students and graduates of their nursing schools, participated actively in saving the lives of the victims. There was a strong collaboration between the white sisters' medical personnel, the few Nigerian sisters and the local people on medical intervention and aid relief (Wall, 2018). St Mary's hospital, established in 1952, had during the war about 150 beds. Many of the Protestants who were white left the country during the civil war, but Medical Missionaries of Mary Catholic Sisters, the Holy Rosary Catholic sisters and many Irish Catholic priests decided to stay behind (Wall, 2018).

The Catholic nuns or sisters, as in the 1930s, could only become nurses and physicians but could not become surgeons, midwives or obstetricians. The Canon Law of the Catholic Church forbade them from working in theatre, and this could be linked to the modesty required of them with their vow of chastity. One of the nuns, Anna Dengel, who worked in India, was very concerned about the Muslim women secluded through purdah. She finally wrote a petition to the Vatican on this, and in 1936, the ban was lifted. The sisters did not just see the need for the sister surgeons and midwives to attend to the needs of women, but also sisters were needed to teach birth control

(Wall, 2018). The sisters and their co-workers worked tirelessly to meet the people's medical, social and spiritual needs during the war.

One could say thanks to the liberation brought by the petition written by Anne Dengel, the nuns were already free to carry out their medical functions fully, and they could give the needed treatment to the victims of the civil war. During the war, sister-nurses, who were almost all white, did practically all that the medical doctors could do. God worked miraculously in the lives of these nuns or sisters during the war. Sometimes they faced difficult situations in which they had to apply wisdom and documentary to remedy the situations since they were the only ones who could attend to such needs. One of those was the case of Sr. Pauline, a paediatrician who had to perform surgeries on adults during the war. When the surgical procedures became challenging and uncertain, she had to read instructions from the surgical textbook as she operated (Wall, 2018).

The Catholic Church in Nigeria established hospitals, maternities and clinics and nursing and midwifery schools for Nigerian students. Around 1962, the Holy Rosary Sisters' Hospital Emekuku and St Luke's Anua schools of nursing and midwifery were the earliest recognised by the Nursing Council of Nigeria and the British General Nursing Council. It was very helpful and significant that Catholic sisters or nuns could offer impressive procedures of modern medicine, such as safer surgery and caesarean sections. This contributed in no small measure to the growth of Nigeria's nursing and medical profession (Schran in Wall, 2018).

After the civil war, the federal government of Nigeria was hostile to the Catholic Church and accused her of prolonging it because she fed and provided healthcare services to their supposed enemies. By this, 300 priests and 200 sisters were expelled from the country, and just a few were recalled in 1970. When the expatriates left, the Nigerian sisters, who had also received adequate training, were administrating those hospitals and healthcare facilities. The government took over some of the hospitals belonging to the Catholic nuns. Some of the sisters who have received adequate training in nursing and medicine were appointed by the government to be in charge of the Catholic hospitals as heads of schools of nursing and midwifery, matrons and deputy matrons (Hastings, 1989). The health intervention of the Catholic Church in Nigeria is more visible in HIV/AIDS control and the management of Ebola virus disease as well as the Covid-19 pandemic.

Catholic Church and Postcolonial Health Interventions: HIV/AIDS Control in Nigeria

The Catholic Church is hierarchical but well-organised. At the national level, there is the bishop liaison that ensures that the health department of the Catholic Secretariat follows the laid-down Catholic ethical behaviours in healthcare delivery; there is also the health secretary who works directly with the health coordinators of all the 58 Catholic dioceses in Nigeria. At the diocesan level, a health coordinator and his team oversee the work at all the health institutions under the diocese. Most often, some poor people cannot pay the little fees that may be charged after treatment. Irrespective of their religion or tribe, if it is established that they cannot pay the fees because of poverty, such people are left to go free without payment. The Catholic Church in Nigeria continues to reach out to the sick in various ways. At the outbreak of any new disease, the Catholic Church positions herself through her structure so that she may not be overwhelmed by the pandemic. For instance, the first cases of HIV/AIDS were observed in Lagos, and Anambra states, respectively, in 1985, with a 13-year-old sexually active girl and a female commercial sex worker from a neighbouring West African Country, which was reported at an international conference in 1986 (Balogun, 2010). Soon after, through her structures, the Catholic Church set up counselling and screening units in almost most of her health facilities to stop the stig-matisation of people living with HIV/AIDS (PLWHA) and the spread of the epidemic. The Church contacted her major partner, Catholic Relief Services (CRS) of the Catholic Bishops' Conference of the USA domicile in Nigeria, which was already working with the Catholic healthcare services in Nigeria, to support testing and the provision of antiretroviral therapy.

The Catholic Relief Services is the brainchild of the United States Confer-ence of Catholic Bishops (USCCB) to respond to the gospel challenge of the love of God and neighbour. As a non-governmental organisation (NGO), it was founded in 1943 to attend to the needs of the survivors of World War II in Europe. Since then, the commission has reached over 130 million people in over 100 countries. The mission of CRS is to support people with low incomes in the United States and disadvantaged people in foreign countries. They work in the spirit of Catholic Social Teaching (CTS) to uphold the sacredness of human life and the dignity of the human person. It defends, protects and advances human life worldwide by directly meeting people's basic needs and advocating solutions to injustices. CRS is a pro-life organisa-tion committed to preserving the sacredness and dignity of human life from conception to natural death. While their mission is entrenched in the Cath-olic faith, their operations serve people exclusively in need, irrespective of race, religion or ethnicity. As the official international humanitarian agency of the Catholic community in the United States of America, CRS is moti-vated by the example of Jesus Christ to ease suffering, provide support and foster charity and justice. CRS shares in humanitarian initiatives engaged in by many other groups, including governments, other faith communities and secular institutions. Though these aforementioned institutions do not always work in line with the full choice of Catholic Social Teaching, the agency still works with them but focuses only on interventions that are in keeping with Catholic social teachings.

CRS began work in Nigeria the year the country gained its independence. In 1967 during the Nigerian Civil War, she worked tirelessly in emergency response. Like other Catholic, bodies (priests and nuns) involved in health and humanitarian activities during the war, they were told to leave the country, and they obliged. They only returned 30 years later, precisely in 2000, after the military rule and during the democratic regime. Their return was at the invitation of the Catholic Bishops Conference of Nigeria (CBCN). Since the return of CRS, it has been working in partnership with the Catholic Church in Nigeria, other faith-based organisations (FBOs), community-based organisations (CBOs), the private sectors, government institutions, local and international NGOs to implement a range of complex programmes, and they get support from different donors and private funds. According to CRS findings, the health indicator of Nigeria is among the poorest in the world. The country was cited as having the second-largest number of people living with HIV worldwide, and it accounts for about 9% of the global HIV epidemic. Because of HIV/AIDS, millions of children have been made orphaned and vulnerable. Again, Nigeria has the highest burden of malaria in the world, and this accounts for the high maternal and childhood illness and death.

Many of their interventions have been around three priority sectors: health system strengthening (HSS), emergency response, agriculture and livelihoods. The health programme addresses HIV/AIDS, nutrition, malaria and routine immunisation for polio eradication and others. They have also provided support to orphans and vulnerable children, and their caregivers. The agency started the intervention on malaria in Nigeria in 2011. It could carry out the programme with the grant it got from Global Funds to Fight AIDS, Tuberculosis and Malaria (GFATM). These malaria interventions address the prevention and the management of malaria at the levels of household, community and health facilities and support the strengthening of Nigeria's malaria health system. Still from the same donors, she was able to access funds to support gender-sensitive HIV/AIDS prevention, care and treatment services by strengthening the quality of health delivered in 127 facilities across Nigeria. The strategy used was mentorship to health facilities, improving laboratory service equipment and promoting effective supply chain management for pharmacy and laboratory supplies. CRS could also access funds from United States Agency for International Development (USAID) to implement two major projects that ended in 2018. The projects were Comprehensive Care for Children (4 Children) and Sustainable Mechanism for Improving Household Empowerment (SMILE). The goal of the projects was to improve access to HIV-sensitive services and support for Orphans and Vulnerable Children (OVC), and their households. Still, on HIV/AIDS, CRS is implementing CDC-funded FASTER (Faith-based Action for Scaling up Testing and Treatment for the Epidemic Response). She collaborates with the government, at the national and state levels, to strengthen paediatric HIV case finding and ensure that HIV-infected children have access to high-quality, age-appropriate clinic care and community-based support.

For the Catholic Church in Nigeria to better organise and coordinate its humanitarian responses, in which health is one of the major focus, in 2010, the Agency, Catholic Caritas Foundation of Nigeria (CCFN), was founded by the Catholic Bishops Conference of Nigeria (CBCN). The CCFN is the specialised Agency of the Church in Nigeria coordinating the development and humanitarian interventions. Their intervention approach has been through projects, outreach, training/workshops, seminars and emergency response to crises leveraging the principles of Catholic Social Teachings. They reach out to the needy persons in the country regardless of their tribe, colour and religious affiliation. An agency that has only operated for about a decade has a record of accomplishment of the increasing number of persons and communities that have benefited from her humanitarian interventions, especially in health and health-related issues.

As explained earlier, the Agency leverages the Catholic Church's existing structure in Nigeria. She serves as the umbrella organisation for all the regional institutions of the church through which the implementation of development-oriented programmes and interventions are made possible. CCFN is a member of Caritas Internationalis, a global confederation of 166 member nations, which share a common mission, and has touched almost every part of the world over the century. She has channelled her interventions, projects and activities through six core thematic areas: emergency and humanitarian response, health and HIV, agriculture and livelihood, good governance, institutional capacity strengthening (ICS) and human trafficking and migration. There are also two silent ones: education and gender; since they are cross-cutting issues, they are embedded in all the six core thematic areas. Our focus in this study is health and HIV.

Health is an important component of the Catholic Church's mandate, and it continues to be the focal point in the activities of Caritas Nigeria since its inception in 2010. This unit promotes every human wellness and integral human development with special emphasis on communicable and noncommunicable diseases and maternal and newborn children. Leveraging on the existing structure of the Catholic Church in Nigeria in implementing her programme, she can pull together tremendous capacities to execute hundreds of primary and secondary health facilities spread across the country. The different programme components of the Agency under health are as follows: Programme Management, Grants, Clinical Care and Treatment, Adherence/Prevention, Laboratory Services, Orphan and Vulnerable Children (OVC), Strategic Information, Pharmacy and Supply Chain Management.

As of March 2023, the Agency has carried out the following interventions: 4,043,535 persons have been tested for HIV. The clients that were being placed in care were 165,787. The positive pregnant women identified were 431,378. The number of positive pregnant mothers identified was 378; 19,040 positive pregnant mothers were placed on Antiretroviral Therapy; 20,271 Early Infant Diagnoses (EID) were carried out. In addition, 3,100 positive clients with tuberculosis (TB) were placed on antiretroviral therapy; 90,006 OVCs have been given care and support; 3,216 healthcare workers, staff and partners were trained; 371 communities and partner institutions in 17 states were impacted.

The Catholic Caritas Foundations has collaborated with many international organisations to implement high-level projects in Nigeria, especially in Health and HIV/AIDS. Barley, a year after registering with the Corporate Affairs Commission, precisely in September 2011, won her first major award in her Health and HIV/AIDS folder called the Sustainable HIV Care and Treatment Action in Nigeria (SUSTAIN). This project, funded by the US President's Emergency Plan for AIDS Relief (PEPFAR), was implemented for five years. Through this project, she carried out a comprehensive HIV care, treatment and prevention programme in 12 states in Nigeria, namely, Benue, Delta Kaduna, Oyo, Ondo, Ogun, Kogi, Nasarawa, Osun, Plateau, Lagos and the Federal Capital Territory (FCT). She was also in collaboration with 141 faith-based health facilities (covering comprehensive centres and stand-alone ante-natal clinics focusing on the prevention of mother-to-child transmission of HIV and 13 community-based organisations) and psycho-social support groups. This collaboration enabled her to execute important activities, including the following: Community Engagement for Demand Creation and Behavioral Change, HIV Testing and Counseling, HIV Treatment, Care and Support, Prevention, Support to Orphans and Vulnerable Children, Laboratory Services, Commodity Logistics Management and Information System, and Strategic Information. The SUSTAIN programme significantly contributes to the institutional capacity of the CCFN, thereby positioning it as one of the foremost organisations that implemented integrated public health programmes on a national scale. Through the programme, the CCFN supported the Nigerian government in hosting, updating and analysing the national data repository for diseases of public health importance. In addition, she helped roll out electronic medical Records for real-time Prevention of Mother to Child Transmission (PMTCT) services in 260 PMTCT sites across 32 Local Government Areas of Nigeria. The HIV/AIDS programme continues to run concurrently with other health programmes of the Catholic Church anchored by the CCFN. Some of the partners (donors) of CCFN are as follows: Global Health Initiative of the University of Nevada Las Vegas, United Nations Programme on AIDS (UNAIDS), U.S. Centers for Diseases Control and Prevention (CDC), U.S. President's Emergency Plan for AIDS Relief (PEPFAR) and Catholic Relief Services.

Catholic Church and Ebola Virus Disease in Nigeria

Following the outbreak of Ebola in West African countries of Guinea, Liberia and Sierra Leone, the Ebola Virus Disease (EVD) finally found its way to the shores of Nigeria. Its first point of call was in Lagos, which is the regional hub for economic, industrial and travel activities, and home to over 21 million people (Egbule, 2015). The Ebola saga started in Lagos on 20 July 2014, when an acutely ill ECOWAS diplomat of Liberian origin travelling from Liberia arrived at the Murtala Mohammed Airport in Lagos. The possibility of an EVD outbreak in Lagos posed a huge epidemiological concern due to its densely populated slums and unsanitary conditions, thus making it a potentially conducive environment for communicable diseases such as EVD to thrive easily (WHO, 2014). Several strategies were quickly deployed to tackle the outbreak, and just as the victory against EVD outbreak in Lagos was in sight, the virus spread to Port Harcourt on 1 August due to a breach in surveillance. Suffice it to say that the index case (Liberian diplomat) infected two ECOWAS associates and health workers at the hospital that attended to him, which led to a cascade of secondary transmission. The EVD outbreak came to an end after three months, with a total of 898 contacts who were linked to the index case, including 351 primary and secondary contacts and 547 tertiary and higher-order contacts. Nigeria confirmed a total of 19 cases, with an average case fatality rate of 40% constituting 7 deaths and 12 survivors (Shuaib et al., 2014).

Nigeria was certified Ebola-free in October 2014, with a total of 894 identified contacts, and about 18,500 persons who were followed up on a day-to-day basis fora duration of 21 days. As at the time of certification, Nigeria had undergone 42 days without any suspected or confirmed case of EVD (WHO, 2014). The laborious efforts of the Nigerian government and other critical stakeholders help to contain the EVD epidemic in Nigeria (Faleye, 2017). The Catholic Church, being aware of the fact that the disease had found its way into Nigeria, began sensitisation of the populace in all her healthcare facilities by even using the pulpit to carry out the sensitisation. Despite the danger inherent in coming in contact with the infected person, she explored ways of reaching out to those infected with EVD through pastoral care. St John Paul II explains the components of pastoral care and the benefits of it on the sick person:

> This activity must be capable of sustaining and fostering attention, nearness, presence, listening, dialogue, sharing, and real help toward individuals in moments when sickness and suffering sorely test not only faith in God and his love as Father. Such pastoral initiatives find most meaningful expression in sacramental celebrations with and for the sick, as a source of strength amid pain and weakness, hope amid despair, and as an occasion of joyful encounter.
>
> (Paul, 1987, n. 54)

This pastoral care include pastoral visit to the sick and praying with them, communicating with the sick persons and re-kindling hope in them, the Catholic priests hearing their confessions, giving them the sacrament of the holy Eucharist, reintegration of the patient who has recovered into the parish community and performing funerals. Knowing how infectious the disease was, not much was done in coming into direct contact with the infected persons except when it was proven safe by the healthcare practitioners. Regarding the funerals, this the Catholic Church did for members who died of the disease since caskets were well sealed and proper guidelines were followed. Prayers were offered for both the infected and the affected. Being an infectious disease and a dreaded one for that matter, the priests helped to re-integrate the survivors back into the church and even into their families.

Catholic Church and COVID-19 Interventions

The coronavirus disease (COVID-19) case was first reported in Nigeria on 27 February 2020 in Ogun State. The government since then made concerted efforts to contain, interrupt and end the transmission of the virus among Nigerians. Knowing that the government could not do it alone, the Catholic Church in Nigeria, through the CCFN, worked with the Message of Hope Steering Committee members and their peers among the different congregations, the relevant government agencies at sub-national levels across the six geo-political regions to raise awareness and acceptance of COVID-19. Added to the intervention of the CCFN in the area of health, the Catholic Bishops Conference of Nigeria (CBCN), in May 2020, offered all 425 health facilities belonging to the Catholic Church across the country as isolation centres for COVID-19 patients. This was in swift response to the federal government's concern over the unavailability of adequate bed spaces to accommodate all COVID-19 patients in the country (Adebowale-Tambe, 2020). Catholic Caritas Foundation carried out many concrete activities during the COVID-19 pandemic. From 3 August to 6 August 2021, there was a COVID-19 Contact Tracing and Management Training for the staff of Caritas Nigeria and the ministries, departments and agencies supporting the Coronavirus Aids Relief and Economic Security (CARES Act) Project at national and state levels. The goal of the exercise was to provide knowledge and skills for effective COVID-19 contact tracing and management. It was also to build capacity on the use of Surveillance, Outbreak Response Management and Analysis System (SORMAS), which was an open response software for COVID-19 surveillance. Thirteen resource persons came to give input on different aspects. These are some of the topics treated: the National COVID-19 Response Strategy, Overview of the CARE Act Project, Basics of COVID-19 Surveillance Contact Tracing Processes, Faith Community Perspective and Response, Presentation of COVID-19 Vaccines, Practicum on the Use of the SORMAS Tool and COVID-19 Testing Option (Including Guidelines and Supplier-Specific Instructions/Diagnostics and Inventory Management). At the end of the training, the participants, numbering about 46, expressed satisfaction over the training they had received and that it was going to increase their knowledge and skills on COVID-19 contact tracing and management and better understanding of data entry, analysis and management using SORMAS software. The trainers in turn went to their various states to carry out the step-down trainings.

Conclusion

The Catholic Church through her healthcare system has been able to reach the hard-to-reach with her mission of caring for the sick and the vulnerable in Nigeria even before the colonial era but most significantly during the postcolonial era. In doing this, she has enjoyed collaboration and financial assistance from the international community to carry out the various projects and programmes. As illustrated by this chapter, the health intervention of the Catholic Church is more visible in HIV/AIDS control and the management of Ebola virus disease as well as the Covid-19 pandemic. Communication and accountability, being key in collaborative ministry especially in healthcare delivery, have helped the church in sustaining her partnership with the different stakeholders. Her resilient spirit has made it possible to move on even when the situations seemed very tough like the experiences during the civil war. Her long-time planning in training and re-training of their staff to carry out multiple tasks like working as orderly at the same time working as interpreters helped in no small measure. With the much interventions the Catholic Church has done in Nigeria, and the much experiences and expertise she has gained over the years, she hopes to continue to reach out to all people since she believes that every human carries the image and likeness of God.

References

Adebowale-Tambe, N. (2020). COVID-19: Catholic Church Donates 425 Health Facilities as Isolation Centres. *Premium Times*. www.premiumtimesng.com/news/top-news/392311-covid-19-catholic-church-donates-425-health-facilities-as-isolation-centres-official.html?tztc=1. Accessed 11 March 2023.

Akindele, F. and Adegbite, W. (1999). *Sociology and Politics of English in Nigeria*. Ile Ife: Obafemi Awolowo University Press.

Balogun, A.S. (2010). HIV/AIDS Epidemic in the History of Nigeria, 1986–2007. *Journal of the Historical Society of Nigeria*, 19: 166–176.

Calvet, L. (1999). *Pour une écologie des langues du monde*. Paris: Plon.

Catholic Caritas Foundation of Nigeria. (2022). HIV/AIDS Programme. www.caritasnigeria.org/. Accessed 11 March 2023.

Catholic Relief Services Nigeria Website. (2023). CRS in Nigeria. www.crs.org/our-work-overseas/where-we-work/nigeria. Accessed 22 March 2023.

Dries, A. (1998). *The Missionary Movement in American Catholic History*. Maryknoll, NY: Orbis Books.

Egbule, J. (2015). A Health Protection Essay on the Outbreak of EBOLA in Nigeria 2014. MSc thesis. Public Health Protection, Faculty of Health and Social Sciences, University of Bedfordshire.

Faleye, O.A. (2017). Sociospatial Networks and Trans-Border Epidemic Surveillance in West Africa: The Ebola Outbreak of 2014–2015 in Perspective. *The Nigerian Health Journal*, 17(3): 61–69.

Hastings, A. (1989). *African Catholicism: Essays in Discovery*. London: SCM Press.

Kant, I. (1996). *The Metaphysics of Morals*. Cambridge and New York: Cambridge University Press.

The Library of Congress Country Studies and CIA World Factbook. (1991). Nigeria History of Modern Medical Services. https://photius.com/countries/nigeria/society/nigeria_society_history_of_modern_me~10005.html. Accessed 28 February 2023.

Paul, J. (1987). *Sollicitudo rei socialis* [Encyclical Letter], 30 December. www.vatican.va/holy_father/john_paul_ii/encyclicals/documents/hf_jp-ii_enc_30121987_sollicitudo-rei-socialis_en.html. Accessed 19 March 2023.

Shuaib, F., Gunnala, R., Musa, E.O., Mahoney, F.J., Oguntimehin, O., Nguku, P.M., et al. (2014). Ebola Virus Disease Outbreak – Nigeria. *MMWR Morbidity and Mortality Weekly Report*, 63(39): 867–872.

Wall, B.M. (2018). Changes in Nursing and Mission in Post-Colonial Nigeria. In *Colonial Caring*. Manchester, UK: Manchester University Press. https://doi.org/10.7765/9781526129369.00015; ResearchGate. www.researchgate.net/publication/327127013_Changes_in_nursing_and_mission_in_post-colonial_Nigeria. Accessed 8 February and 28 February 2023.

World Health Organization. (2014). Nigeria Is Now Free of Ebola Virus Transmission. www.who.int/mediacentre/news/ebola/20-october-2014/en/index1.html. Accessed 11 March 2022.

Part III

Socio-Political Significance of Sexuality, Medicaments, and Sexually Transmitted Diseases

7 Socio-Political Significance of Asian Aphrodisiacs and African Sexualities in Postcolonial Zimbabwe

Basure S. Hardlife

Introduction

This chapter focuses on socio-political significance of the consumption of alternative medicines in postcolonial Zimbabwe. There seems to be a growing niche market for the sale and consumption of unconventional medicines which usually claim to deal with those problems which have largely escaped medicalization. The problems appear to be trivialized or fail to receive due attention for several reasons. The hidden nature of sexual behaviour is also fertile ground for the propagation of unquestioned claims and myths, something which has seen numerous elixirs of sexual performance being peddled. The shame, mystery, and secrecy surrounding sexual behaviour has resulted in the growth of underground economies of knowledge and products meant to bring about solutions to various sexual issues ranging from underperformance, sexually transmitted infections, sexual expectations to even relationships. It is against this background that this chapter examines knowledge and practices surrounding alternative medical practices and sexualities in postcolonial Zimbabwe. The chapter exploits data from ethnographic fieldwork conducted mainly in the city of Masvingo in Zimbabwe, while also drawing insights from broader networks which link respondents in the city with clients and suppliers within and outside the country.

Alternative Medicine, Informality, and the Regulation of Healing

Medical consumption is one of the most regulated arenas of public life. The production, distribution, and consumption of medicinal products must go through rigorous testing and comply with different sets of global and local health laws and standards. However, the legislation of medicine on the other hand has fuelled the growth of an underworld of medicines, characterized by counterfeits, banned substances as well as products of questionable efficacy especially in relation to the claims that are associated with these products. The adherence to laws, regulations, and standards should be seen as the backbone of the designation of the medicines understudy as 'alternative medicines'. Whereas some would see the term 'alternative' as a deviation

DOI: 10.4324/9781003429135-11

from the conventional and biomedical medicines, it should be noted that everything surrounding these medicines is of an alternative nature. They are characterized by alternative ways of distribution, which cuts off the specialist physician and pharmacist and upgrades the ordinary person to become both the physician and the pharmacist. They are also characterized by alternative philosophies, often deviating from the formalized medical knowledge, in favour of religious, mythical, traditional, and pseudoscientific claims. They tell of phantastic places and stories about utopian places, faraway places, and valiant journeys and escapades of those who would have used or consumed the medicines. In this chapter, most of the medicines which are discussed are often linked to Asian origins, something which influenced me to coin the term Asian Inspired Complementary and Alternative Medicine (AICAM) (Basure, 2021). This type of alternative medicine seems to be flooding the contemporary markets of alternative medicines.

Historically alternative medicine can be seen to be an outcome of the superimposition of Western medical systems through colonial conquest (Lowes and Montero, 2018). The colonial masters implemented their own medical systems which were deeply rooted in the Western cultural systems. The biomedical model assumed the role of mainstream medicine, in line with biomedical standards. Colonialism informalized any other form of knowledge in medicine (Daffé et al., 2021). The outcome can be seen in the contemporary dichotomy which puts biomedical knowledge on one side while treating every other form of medical knowledge as the 'other'. In this otherized section, numerous healing claims can be found which include traditional medicine as well as numerous forms of quackery and snake oil peddling (Bigliardi, 2019). This arena has been trivialized and – like a mad man – has not been accorded any space within the discourses of modern healing. Hence, this chapter notes that in order to have a holistic public health approach, it is imperative to cast eyes even on these trivialized approaches to medicine since they have numerous impacts on people's health-seeking behaviours. Some of the effects include reluctance to seek specialist assistance, a suspicious and sceptic attitude towards the public health system, characterized by a mistrust of conventional medicine, as well as the potential danger posed by the consumption of unregulated and unstandardized medicines.

Though different forms of healing knowledge have been informalized, studies have shown that folk knowledge and alternative medicine are the first port of call when it comes to people's health-seeking behaviour (Chavhunduka, 1998; Ernst, 2000; Ernst and Fugh-Berman, 2002; Siahpush, 1999). Public health systems are often inaccessible and riddled with stigma such that people seek the easier way out. The private and unstandardized nature of alternative systems makes them more attractive for patients, though at times the benefits of such systems have always been subject to ambiguity and contention. They lie in the arena of the unproven and rely mainly on personal testimony to establish the efficacy of such medical products. However, using the informal channels, knowledge, and medical information travel faster through people's social networks.

The Postcolonial Condition and Medical Power Dynamics

Whereas the history of modern public health discourse has undeniably been shaped by coloniality, the postcolonial conditions are increasingly influencing the nature and character of public health (Lang, 2001; Ramos et al., 2022). Postcoloniality implies the dismantling of anything colonial and a general movement away from the discriminatory and anti-African attitudes of the colonial system (Packard, 2020; Packard et al., 2003). This has also meant that embracing alternative medicines can be interpreted as a form of resistance to colonialism. In line with Michel Foucault's postulations on biopolitics (Means, 2022), public health approaches have often been viewed as cementing state power, whereas resistance to these could be interpreted as constituting a reclamation of that power (Villella, 2022). The abuse of power at the local or global level often found expression in genocidal policies which Achille Mbembe conceptualized as necropolitcs (Mbembe, 2003, 2019). The inequality in the global political economy of development impacts global health. For instance, the Look East Policy and its associated influx of Asian Aphrodisiac and its deleterious effects on Zimbabweans constitute a coloniality of medicaments and sexuality in the South-South cooperation.

In Zimbabwe, the postcolonial narrative seek to decolonise Western ideas that are seen as evil and dominating through neocolonialism (Mararike, 2019). Hence, the rejection of anything Western can signify victory over colonialism. The anti-Western narrative has often been coupled with an embrace of Asian partnership, encapsulated in the government's Look East Policy (Ojakorotu and Kamidza, 2018). This can explain the influx of Asian products, merchandise, and medicines which I have bundled under the term AICAM. In this vein, the political ideologies cannot be divorced from the public health domain. It determines issues such as accreditation, testing and licensing of medicinal products as well as policing and surveillance on the usage of these medicines. One interesting experience of the postcolonial ideological warfare in Zimbabwe was the refusal by the state to allow the use of Western COVID-19 vaccines, whilst the Chinese manufactured drugs became the major drug of choice during the state's compulsory vaccination drive (Murewanhema and Dzinamarira, 2022; Suzuki and Yang, 2022). Hence, political ideologies are important in shaping the nature and direction of public health processes. There is an evident soft approach of dealing with products from the East due to the political inclination of the state towards the East.

Sexual Health and Public Health

Sexual health is one of the most problematic areas of public health. This is due to several factors which include the cultures of silence surrounding sexual and reproductive health issues as well as the shame and stigma which accompany discussions of sexual matters in most cultures (Hall, 2020; Marais, 2019). This implies that most individuals explore the terrain of sexual health on their own, with limited assistance coming from circles of trust and friends, whose expertise is also questionable. Hall (2020) further notes a general tendency towards avoiding the exploration of subjects on sexuality within biomedicine. This has meant that a veil remains which treat sexual issues as sacrosanct and not easily a subject of choice in both academic studies as well as the field of health and healing. Measures to deal with reproductive health problems have not been quite comprehensive since they have focused more on dealing with issues along the biomedical model. Public health focus on sexual health has been limited to addressing different sexually transmitted ailments, while other arenas of sexuality such as pleasure have generally been ignored (Ford et al., 2019). This has left a glaring gap which alternative medicine has gladly occupied. All sorts of remedies to enhance sexual pleasure and expectations are sold on the alternative medicine markets. This is also coupled with beauty enhancement products, which are meant to transform people's physical appearance to satisfy a variety of sexual fantasies.

Most AICAM traders in the area under study have come up with what they term natural herbal solutions to addressing sexual needs. There is an implicit assumption that if the products are 'natural' then they are side effects-free, hence individuals do not hesitate to consume these alternative medical remedies. However, studies have shown that most of these purported natural remedies are actually falsified drugs since they contain undeclared chemical components which give people the desired results (Yéléhé-Okouma et al., 2021). Some 'natural' sexual enhancements have been found to contain chemicals such as sildenafil, and these chemicals are often present in unregulated quantities since there is little or no oversight on the manufacturing and selling processes (Yéléhé-Okouma et al., 2021). Addressing sexual pleasure should therefore be part and parcel of public health programming since this arena has been neglected, thereby influencing the mushrooming of practices which put people at risk. Some of the respondents I interviewed who had consumed sexual enhancements from alternative medicine dealers reported various negative effects though they never sought medical attention. These ranged from dizziness, splitting headaches, prolonged erections, to bloodshot eyes. One respondent noted that he experienced a severe headache while he could feel pressurized veins which were visible on his face. However, this did not deter him from using the drug as he felt that it gave him the desired results despite the side effects. As the respondent puts it:

> Now I have been told a trick when you use these *pills* (sexual enhancement pills), you need to drink lots of water and avoid taking the whole pill at once. Rather break it into three or four portions.

Thus, fulfilling sexual pleasure was more important than the health risk posed by unverified medicines touted as 'natural pills'. Hence, most people may be at risk from consuming untested substances while they put their trust in the claim that these are natural products. The side effects of the products are just seen as normal experiences which can be dealt with as long as the individual experienced the required sexual arousal and pleasure. The focus on the end goal of excellent sexual performance points to a generation fixated on sexualities.

The Sexual Revolution, Heightening Sexualities

Postcolonial Zimbabwe has been characterized by mixed feelings towards sexualities. While there seems to be control and regulation of some elements of sexuality, one arena which is difficult to pin down is the issue of sexual pleasure. This is a hidden and private space, far removed from the scrutiny of the public eye and regulation. However, that which is often hidden often manifests in the public sphere through unconventional means. Sexual satisfaction, though it resides in the hidden private sphere, is increasingly becoming a public topic of discussion, such that one can observe that we are in the midst of a sexual revolution, characterized by an insatiable focus on sexual performance and satisfaction. Coupled with the digital revolution, people have found ways to discuss and offer all sorts of solutions and experiences in relation to sexual performance (Muwonwa, 2021). It is on these platforms that you find AICAM traders also bringing in their merchandise to contribute to the discourse on sexual performance. As one message advertising sexual supplements in Zimbabwe read:

> Save yourself from the embarrassment of being useless in bed, imagine she starts cheating because you can't satisfy her well, think about it!! Hit to her satisfaction and she will never leave you or look next-door!

Such kinds of messaging capture the prevalent focus on sexual performance. It is also the subject of private discussions among friends and colleagues. And through these networks, communities of sexual practice are created, with links, information, and of course herbal supplements to enhance the game. As the excerpt from a conversation shows:

> My brother, can you pass by, there is a certain coffee which I have I want you to go and try it. It's so effective. If you are not sure ask John, I gave him last week and he called me speechless about how it worked for him. I want you to have it, then you will come back and tell me what you are going to experience.

Those were the words of one of my long-time acquaintances in the city encouraging me to test the efficacy of a sex-enhancing coffee which he had just acquired from his networks. Not that I had complained to him about any sexual performance, but his desire for me to also experience what he had experienced. Such is the increase in attention towards sexual issues which have become so prevalent in contemporary urban spaces. There is a general belief in increased sexual performance, something which perhaps may be an outcome of media and internet obsession with sexual issues (Muwonwa, 2021). It has become commonplace to find fliers, street hawkers, and shops selling sexual performance-enhancing paraphernalia. From virginity restoration, sexual performance boosters, to penis enlargement pills and creams, hip and buttock enhancement medicines, we live in a highly sexualized society, with utopian sexual expectations. Sexual masculinities and femininities are continuously being remodelled and reshaped within alternative medicine.

Whereas in the developed world, there has been a steady rise of people who go through the knife to enhance their appearance, the prohibitive costs of such surgery have meant that most of the people in the developing world try to achieve the same results through unconventional medicines and substances. Alternative medicines are viewed as an easier way for individuals to achieve the elements of modern sexual desire. Sexualities are increasingly being expressed, modified, and presented through different redefinitions of masculinities and femininities. For women, the body has also been a site of enhancement to fulfil sexual desire. Well-shaped women are idolized to such an extent that contemporary femininities have pushed most women to do something about their bodies. Moreover, there is a growing expectation for women to also perform in ways which capture their men's attention. Against this backdrop a plethora of remedies ranging from 'Indian sweets' which are said to 'marinate' the female body to increase sensation and sexual satisfaction to other substances such as yoni powder which is said to increase body heat are some of the new products which are redefining sexual experience in Zimbabwe. There is pressure for both men and women to create extraordinary sexual experiences. This in turn fuels a reliance on medicinal aids to ensure that individuals transcend the limitations of their natural bodies. Heightened sexualities should be seen as a motivating factor in the growth of an alternative medicine sector which deals with enhancing sexual experience.

Repackaging Femininities and Masculinities

The expression of maleness and femaleness are increasingly coming under a sexual gaze in contemporary times. Coupled with traditional expectations, individuals are increasingly finding ways to cheat the system and conform to the idealized standards of maleness and femaleness. One such product has been the virginity restoration soaps and kits which have been popular, with women attempting to deceive their partners on sexual purity. Bridal kits, which make one mimic a first sexual encounter, are sold to people who attempt to keep good reputations of sexual purity. Traditionally, in Zimbabwe, virginity signified the value of a woman, with a cow being paid to the in-laws as gratitude for providing a virgin bride (Shenjere-Nyabezi, 2022). The lack of that cow was not only a financial loss but caused embarrassment to the bride's family as this could be interpreted as a failure to properly bring up a child with respectable manners (Matunhu et al., 2019). In contemporary times, online social media platforms often carry interesting perspectives on issues such as virginity, with some users advocating toxic forms of masculinities and femininities. Cults which deride sexual laxity find huge followership among young adults, showing a mutation of sexual purity expectations, especially among women. The value of women is seen to lie in her sexual purity, signified by the concept of virginity. Loss of virginity is seen as loss of value, which significantly jeopardizes one's pool of potential marriage suitors.

Moreover, physical beauty, interpreted through facial appearance and physical body structure, often seen through a perverted focus on erogenous zones and sexualized female bodies, can be seen to be instrumental in pushing individuals to seek ways to enhance themselves. As noted earlier, individuals try to improve their sexual performance by improving sexual appeal through body-altering substances. These include skin-lightening products, and body parts transforming substances such as pill and herbs to enhance the hips or buttocks. Men also are seen dabbling with concoctions for penis enlargement, something which point to a masculinity based upon sexual prowess. This poses a significant public health challenge as people consume different alternative medical products which come into the country labelled as dietary supplements or herbal medicines.

The Trade and Distribution of Alternative Sexual Enhancements

The distribution of alternative medical products follows an elaborate web of local and international networks of individuals, some mostly who pursue profit motives. Technology and online platforms are also at the centre of this web since it facilitates the whole process from distribution to marketing of the products. Most of the individuals interviewed noted that online platforms were important in connecting the manufacturers with the distributors and subsequently the distributors and the consumers. In Zimbabwe, the economic challenges facing most people have forced them to go into petty capitalism, where they sell anything and everything just to get a little profit. One of the fast-moving products of this trade can be seen to be these sexual-enhancement products since they most often find a ready market and people purchase them often. There are several small shops, usually characterized by many traders tightly packed in one room as they try to cut down on rental charges. Such shops contain most of these foreign alternative medicines which claim to deal with a variety of ailments, including sexual problems, using natural ingredients. It is also common to find these products on the streets as well as on glass cabinets inside salons and barber shops. These medicines are continually changing the urban landscape and constituting part of most of the backyard urban shops. However, those who command more resources have had the ability to rent bigger spaces where they operate in a manner which mimic biomedical clinics. One would find people who perform the role of the nurse as well as others who will be operating like the biomedical doctor.

Apart from established shops, most of the trade in AICAM products followed individualized networks, while some even relied on pyramid-scheme-like systems where one sold and recruited others to sell products so that they could increase commission (Hornberger, 2019). These often use brochures, which act as manuals, where they simply read preset symptoms and dispense prepacked medicines. As one of my key informants noted:

> I am a member of an international health organization with our head-quarters in Malaysia. All our products come from Malaysia and are shipped through South Africa. However, you cannot buy directly since there are regional consultants for each area, so for me I contact our regional consultant based in South Africa. There are special prices at every level so that everyone gets a profit and the higher you go the better the profits.

The distribution of alternative medical products follows elaborate patterns of global social networks which bring together individuals in different parts of the world. Most of the products which were distributed were not subjected to scrutiny by the regulating authority, that is, the Medicine Control Authority of Zimbabwe (MCAZ). However, some had taken the longer route of seeking clearance, but their registration did not refer to them as medicines but herbal supplements instead. The bulk of AICAM products follow illicit trade routes, where they are smuggled into the country. Most of the distributors of the products testified that they never ran into problems with regulating authorities since there have not been any visits to check the products they sell. However, the only regulation came from city council officials who try to clamp down on illegal vending and prohibited usage of space. The regulatory capacity of state agencies is questionable, as well as their capacity to success-fully test substances to establish the safety of products.

Whereas some may try to look at the health dimension of this global trade, it is quite evident that the profit motive permeates most of this trade. Most of the people interviewed showed that this trade was their major income earner, while others engaged in the practice as a side hustle which improves their cashflows. Hence individual traders focus on those products which bring the most returns as they are driven by the desire to improve their incomes. The postcolonial vagaries of economic lack create conditions which force individuals to engage in penny capitalism or what Jeremy Jones (2010) called *kukiyakiya* (making do). From the capital, Harare, to other smaller cities, there is an overwhelming presence of individuals trading in these sexual enhancements as people attempt to eke out a living in a harsh economic environment. Some of the respondents who engaged in the sale of AICAM products included civil servants, including those who worked in the health sector. The majority testified that the proceeds of the trade were lucrative and worth the effort as they significantly contributed to household income.

Apart from the common claims to heal difficult and chronic conditions, sex-related products dominate the distribution of AICAM. These included substances mentioned before like *yoni* powder, which was said to be important for women as it could tighten and increase the heat, something which improved sexual performance. There were also several substances which were thought to improve sensation and even sometimes spiritually lock a partner to ensure faithfulness or to increase the love bond. Most of the products also had elaborate philosophies which constituted part of their ideologies of healing. Some claimed that their herbs work by cleansing the body and restoring its balance and thereby improving sexual performance. Others added a spiritual and magical dimension where one was expected to influence the behaviour of their partner through the consumption of the medicines.

Alternative Medicine and Aphrodisiacs: Public Health Implications

Though most people may attest to achieving their desired results through the usage of imported alternative medicine, one cannot ascertain the ingredients and safety of the substances since they are never subjected to independent scrutiny. Cases where prominent politicians succumbed to death during sexual encounters may also point to the questionable nature of these sexual AICAM, especially where there is no specified dosage. Hence there is a potential of individuals exposing themselves to future health complications, even medical emergencies, due to this unchecked consumption of unverifiable medicines. Apart from these evident fatalities, there are potential long-term effects which may not be possible to measure at the present.

There was a notable relationship between medical scepticism and the consumption of AICAM as most people who subscribed to these medicines were also highly likely to believe medical conspiracy theories. Hence the domain of AICAM consumption is also riddled with disinformation and misinformation which may significantly alter people's health-seeking patterns. This creates an urgent need for measures to counter disinformation and ensure that individuals receive proper medical advice. The third public health issue which is evident in the study is the practicality of policing the usage and consumption of alternative medicines. Most of the AICAM products prevalent in Zimbabwe treaded carefully on the thin line of medical policing and legislations. When it came to registration of products, most were categorized as 'herbal supplements' which were not subject to strict scrutiny, and at the same time people were left to use their discretion when purchasing these products. On the other hand, the marketing and salespeople did not use this language of herbal supplements but instead vigorously marketed their products as biomedical products.

Hence, there is a need to enforce measures which ensure that consumers are not vulnerable to false advertising and ensure that products are sold in relation to the given licenses. The abuse of political ideologies to further the profit motive and distribution of unproven medicines should also be kept in check. Policy making and policing in relation to AICAM remains problematic also due to the micro nature of the trade in the products. Mostly people exploit circles of trust and social networks to convey messages and to sell these products. Transnational links also exist which unite manufacturers and sellers into elaborate webs of business relationships. Moreover, the advent of technology and social media has made it much easier to market and distribute products outside the purview of the law. The last important public health implication of the study should be seen in the focus on sexual pleasure. The study reiterates observations by different scholars that there is a missing dimension when it comes to sexual and reproductive health. Though diseases are addressed, and drugs as well as preventive measures are given attention in sexual health matters, the continued silence on sexual pleasure poses a significant danger to individuals as they are left to navigate this issue in an individual and private manner. This exposes individuals to information and products which may be dangerous and can jeopardize their health in the future. There is need for further study and regulation of this arena to safeguard people and ensure that they are protected from adverse actions which affect their health.

Although it is unfair to blanket alternative medical products, it is important to ensure that these products meet minimum safety guidelines and are subjected to normal processes regulating medical paraphernalia. The usage of herbal and dietary supplements has been noted to be a loophole through which drug falsification occurs. Some scholars advocate the treatment of all dietary supplements as adulterated products until proven otherwise as a measure to ensure that the public is not exposed to drug falsification (Yéléhé-Okouma et al., 2021). The unregulated influx of these dangerous medicaments is an abuse of power at the local and global levels brought about by the inequality in the global political economy of development. Hence there is a need for stricter scrutiny of these products which also calls for enhancing the capacity of local regulatory authorities in a globalized world.

Conclusion

The chapter has put forward several propositions in relation to the experiences and consumption of AICAM products, especially in the context of sexual health. As the adage goes, 'sex sells', the chapter has shown how linking AICAM products to issues of sex and sexual health has been a strategy employed in marketing the products. This local sexual drive has been exploited by dominant powers in the global political economy. Indeed, the inequality in the global political economy of development impacts global health. This is the case of the Look East Policy and its associated influx of Asian Aphrodisiac and its deleterious effects on Zimbabweans. This constitutes a coloniality of medicaments and sexuality in the South-South cooperation. Indeed, political, socio-economic, and cultural factors can all be seen to converge in producing a discourse of the sale and consumption of

AICAM products. Sexual cultures which have commoditized sex and created fetish cults around sexual practice influence a growth in alternative ways of fulfilling the sexual script. Moreover, postcoloniality has given space to previously muffled voices, thereby resulting in the explosion of alternative ways of addressing health issues. Economically, the rise of penny capitalism coupled with economic shocks which have pushed most people to be entrepreneurs have meant that there is a continued presence of individuals willing to engage in the sale of AICAM products. It should be noted that there is relative silence in relation to the policing of alternative medicinal products since they fall under a grey regulatory zone. There are severe public health implications which flow from the relative absence of control of the sale and consumption of sexually linked alternative medicines. The chapter concludes by underscoring the need to review and ensure that practices in the field of complementary medicine are not detrimental to public health, through proper ordering and oversight on the sale of alternative medicines.

References

Basure, H.S. (2021). *In Search of a Cure: Experiences in Alternative Medicine in Masvingo Urban, Zimbabwe*. Doctoral Dissertation, University of Pretoria, Pretoria.

Bigliardi, S. (2019). The Advocates of Pseudoscience Are Not Monsters – But Pseudoscience Is. *Skeptical Inquirer*, 43(6): 58–60.

Chavhunduka, G.L. (1998). *The Professionalization of Traditional Medicine in Zimbabwe*. Harare: Jongwe Printers.

Daffé, Z.N., Guillaume, Y., and Ivers, L.C. (2021). Anti-Racism and Anti-Colonialism Praxis in Global Health – Reflection and Action for Practitioners in US Academic Medical Centers. *The American Journal of Tropical Medicine and Hygiene*, 105(3): 557.

Ernst, E. (2000). Prevalence of Use of Complementary/Alternative Medicine: A Systematic Review. *Bulletin of the World Health Organization*, 78(2): 258–266.

Ernst, E. and Fugh-Berman, A. (2002). Complementary and Alternative Medicine: What Is It All About? *Occupational and Environmental Medicine*, 59(2): 140–144. https://doi.org/10.1136/oem.59.2.140.

Ford, J.V., Vargas, E.C., Finotelli, Jr., I., Fortenberry, J.D., Kismödi, E., Philpott, A., Rubio-Aurioles, E., and Coleman, E. (2019). Why Pleasure Matters: Its Global Relevance for Sexual Health, Sexual Rights and Wellbeing. *International Journal of Sexual Health*, 31(3): 217–230. https://doi.org/10.1080/19317611.2019.1654587.

Hall, L.A. (2020). The Sexual Body. In Cooter, R. and Pickstone, J. (Eds.), *Medicine in the Twentieth Century* (pp. 261–275). London, Taylor & Francis.

Hornberger, J. (2019). Who Is the Fake One Now? Questions of Quackery, Worldliness and Legitimacy. *Critical Public Health*, 29(4): 484–493.

Jones, J.L. (2010). "Nothing Is Straight in Zimbabwe": The Rise of the kukiya-kiya Economy 2000–2008. *Journal of Southern African Studies*, 36(2): 285–299.

Lang, T. (2001). Public Health and Colonialism: A New or Old Problem? *Journal of Epidemiology & Community Health*, 55(3): 162–163.

Lowes, S.R. and Montero, E. (2018). The Legacy of Colonial Medicine in Central Africa. *American Economic Review*, 111(4): 1284–1314.

Marais, K. (2019). Calls for Pleasure: How African Feminists Are Challenging and Unsilencing Women's Sexualities. *Agenda*, 33(3): 87–95.

Mararike, M. (2019). *Zimbabwe Will Never Be a Colony Again! Sanctions and Anti-Imperialist Struggles in Zimbabwe*. Bamenda: Langaa RPCIG.

Matunhu, V., Matunhu, J., and Kalunta-Crumpton, A. (2019). Obtrusive Forms of Violence Against Young Women in Zimbabwe. *Violence against Women of African Descent: Global Perspectives*, 51–72. London: Lexington Books.

Mbembe, J.A. (2003). Necropolitics. *Public Culture*, 15(1): 11–40.

Mbembe, J.A. (2019). *Necropolitics*. Durham: Duke University Press.

Means, A.J. (2022). Foucault, Biopolitics, and the Critique of State Reason. *Educational Philosophy and Theory*, 54(12): 1968–1969.

Murewanhema, G. and Dzinamarira, T. (2022). The COVID-19 Pandemic: Public Health Responses in Sub-Saharan Africa. *International Journal of Environmental Research and Public Health*, 19(8): 4448.

Muwonwa, N. (2021). "Subverting Controls": Historicising the Multi-dimensions of Female Youth Sexuality in Post-colonial Zimbabwe. In *Fending for Ourselves: Youth in Zimbabwe, 1980–2020* (p. 158). Harare, Weaver Press.

Ojakorotu, V. and Kamidza, R. (2018). Look East Policy: The Case of Zimbabwe – China Political and Economic Relations since 2000. *India Quarterly*, 74(1): 17–41.

Packard, R.M. (2020). Post-Colonial Medicine. In *Medicine in the Twentieth Century* (pp. 97–112). London, Taylor & Francis.

Packard, R.M., Cooter, R., and Pickstone, J. (2003). Post-Colonial Medicine. In *Companion to Medicine in the Twentieth Century* (pp. 97–112). London, Taylor & Francis.

Ramos, J.G.P., Garriga-López, A., and Rodríguez-Díaz, C.E. (2022). How Is Colonialism a Sociostructural Determinant of Health in Puerto Rico? *AMA Journal of Ethics*, 24(4): 305–312.

Shenjere-Nyabezi, P. (2022). Ethnoarchaeology of Cattle in Zimbabwe and Surrounds. *Oxford Research Encyclopedia of Anthropology*. https://doi.org/10.1093/acrefore/9780190854584.013.529.

Siahpush, M. (1999). Why Do People Favour Alternative Medicine? *Australian and New Zealand Journal of Public Health*, 23(3): 266–271.

Suzuki, M. and Yang, S. (2022). Political Economy of Vaccine Diplomacy: Explaining Varying Strategies of China, India, and Russia's COVID-19 Vaccine Diplomacy. *Review of International Political Economy*, 30: 1–26.

Villella, P.B. (2022). Disputing Epidemics, Public Health, and Alternative Therapies in Latin American History. *Latin American Research Review*, 57(1): 213–225.

Yéléhé-Okouma, M., Pape, E., Humbertjean, L., Evrard, M., El Osta, R., Petitpain, N., Gillet, P., El Balkhi, S., and Scala-Bertola, J. (2021). Drug Adulteration of Sexual Enhancement Supplements: A Worldwide Insidious Public Health Threat. *Fundamental & Clinical Pharmacology*, 35(5): 792–807.

8 Mass Media, Sexuality and the Social Determinants of HIV/AIDS in Nigeria

Andrew Ate, Ewomazino D. Akpor, and Anthonia I. Otsupius

Introduction

The mass media which comprise radio, television, newspapers, magazines, books andinternet have the ability and capacity to reduce the spread of HIV/AIDS in terms of education and public awareness campaigns. However, the same mass media are seen as instruments for promotion of sexuality leading to HIV/AIDS. Experts confirm this development in different studies. It is noted that uncontrolled exposure of mass media and internet could negatively influence sexual patterns and behaviour of youths (Asekun-Olarinmoye et al., 2014). It has been noted that adolescents use the media as sources of information about sex, drugs, AIDS and violence as well as learn how to behave in relationship (Gruber and Grube, 2000). It is argued further that adolescents face the risk of sexually transmitted infections including HIV/AIDS. These risks are increased by social change and modernization and communication revolutions such as access to cybercafés, pornographic materials and of course exposure to foreign culture through satellite television programmes (Nworgu, 2020).

The power of the mass media to influence sexuality especially among the youths in Nigeria cannot be underestimated. Indeed, the influence of the media portrayals of sexual attitudes and normative expectations of young people is at critical development stage of public health concern (Asekun-Olarinmoye et al., 2014).

HIV is the virus that causes AIDS. It is known as Human Immunodeficiency Virus. Acquired Immune Deficiency Syndrome (AIDS) was a clinical entity in the USA by 1981 and soon after the causative agent was isolated and identified as Human Immunodeficiency Virus (HIV). It is most commonly spread through sexual relationships with infected persons (Amanze, 2006: 101). There are approximately 38 million people across the globe with HIV/AIDS in 2019. Out of these, 36.2 million were adults, while 1.8 million were children (UNAIDS, 2020). Statistics have shown that Nigeria is third in the number of HIV epidemics worldwide (Oladele et al., 2020). UNAIDS (2019) notes that new survey results indicate that Nigeria has an HIV prevalence of 1.4% among adults aged 15–49. The south-south zone has the highest

DOI: 10.4324/9781003429135-12

prevalence at (3.1%), followed by north-central zone, (2.0%) and south-east zone (1.9%). In Nigeria, HIV prevalence is lower in south-west zone (1.1%), the north-east Zone, (1.1%) and the north-west zone (0.6%).

The United States has been a major financier of HIV/AIDS control efforts in Nigeria. Oladele et al. (2020: 2) note that "since 2006, about US $ 4 billion has been spent on HIV control efforts in Nigeria. About 80% of these funds have been from donors-mainly the US President's Emergency Plan for AIDS Relief (PEPFAR) and the Global Fund to fight AIDS Tuberculosis and Malaria (The Global Fund). Firms and households contributed about 0%–2%, with the rest of the funds provided by the Nigerian government". All these efforts were geared towards stemming the tide of HIV/AID in Nigeria. In terms of communication, both the mainstream media and social media have been deployed to disseminate information on HIV/AIDS to people in Nigeria. This study looks at the relationship between mass media, sexuality and HIV/AIDS. It evaluates media offerings that promote sexuality and HIV/AIDS in Nigeria, analyses types of media that lead to the promotion of sexuality and HIV/AIDS in Nigeria and investigates the extent to which mass media promotion of sexuality can lead to HIV/AIDS in Nigeria.

Conceptual Clarifications

Mass media has been described as a means of communication that operates on a large scale, reaching and involving virtually everyone in a society to a greater or lesser degree. Media is plural of medium, which means a channel or vehicle through which something is carried or transmitted. In order words, mass media are channels of communication in modern society primarily the print and electronic media (McQuail, 2000). Mass media can be broadly classified into two: the print media and electronic media. The classification is carried out according to the mechanism involved (Ate, 2008). Under the print media family, we have newspapers, books, magazines, pamphlets, comics and so on. Under broadcast, we have radio, television, motion pictures, videos recordings and so on. Today, with media convergence, the new media (internet) and the social media structures are gradually fusing into the mass media in terms of some operations. Defluer et al. cited by Ate (2008: 63) see the mass media as "devices for moving messages across distances or time to accomplish mass communication". Other experts – Murphy (1997), Dennis (1991) and McQuail (2000) – attest to the power and influence of the mass media in the lives of people and institutions. Sexuality has to do with organized and systematic relationship between people of diverse sexual orientations. The World Health Organization (WHO) (2006) defines sexuality as a

> [c]entral aspect of being human throughout life encompasses sex, gender identities and roles, sexual orientation, exoticism, pleasure, intimacy and reproduction. Sexuality is experienced and expressed in thoughts, fantasies, desires, beliefs, attitudes, values, behaviours, practices, roles

and relationships. While sexuality can include all these dimensions, not all of them are always experienced or expressed. Sexuality is influenced by interaction of biological, psychological, social economic, political, cultural, legal, historical, religious and spiritual factors.

(UNESCO's International Technical Guide of
Sexuality Education, 2018)

UNESCO (2018: 69) affirms that "human beings are born with the capacity to enjoy their sexuality throughout their life". The European Expert Group on Sexuality Education (2015), underscoring the importance of sexuality education, notes that it does not encourage children and young people to have sex but rather strengthens the ability of children and young people to make conscious, satisfying, healthy and respectful choices regarding relationships, sexuality and emotional physical health. There appears to be a connection between the media and sexuality. The mainstream mass media (television, magazines, movies, music and the Internet) provide increasingly frequent portrayers of sexuality (Brown, 2002). The agenda setting theory proposes that "the public agenda or what kinds of things people discuss, think and worry about (Sometimes ultimately press for legislation about) is powerfully shaped and directed by what news media choose to publicize". Wimmer and Dominick contend that agenda setting research examines "the relationship between media priorities and audience priorities in the relative importance of news topic" (Wimmer and Dominick, 2000: 388). It is argued that "mass media have the ability to transfer the salient items on their news agenda to the public agenda" Griffin (2000: 27). The theory is relevant to the study because the mass media can bring to the front burner aspects of sexuality issues or stuff that it wants to sell to the public. By way of drawback, this theory has been criticized on the grounds that past agenda setting studies have neglected possible effects on what people think concerning *who* is important, *where* important things happen and *why* things are important (Davis and Robinson, 1989).

Uses and gratification theory propounded by Katz (1959) probes what Griffin (2012: 358) calls "what people do with the media". The theory has sentenced into oblivion the magic bullet theory which made the media decide what people consume (Ate and Chukwu, 2020). The theory attempts to make sense of the fact that people consume a dazzling array of media messages for all sorts of reasons, and the effect of a given message is unlikely to be the same for everyone (Griffin, 2012). This shows the place of mass media as a social tool of sexuality with implications for sexual health in society. This theory is apt for this study because media offerings with sexual appeals are consumed by the audience because of pleasure and extreme gratification. Garlick (2011), speaking with the American Society in mind, noted that sex is used to sell everything in the country, from liquor to political candidates to automobiles to Tupperware products; in pornography, at least sex is honestly selling itself. What motivates porn consumers according to Guy (1985) is that pornographic movies nowadays begin with the action: a man and a woman appear on the screen and are already fooling around. Experts observe that cross-sectional surveys have found that frequent exposure to sexual media content is associated with increased reports of intentions to have sex, light sexual behaviour (kissing, holding hands) and heavy sexual behaviour, such as intercourse (Ward et al., 2016). Hence, the mass media is an important platform to curb HIV/AIDS in Nigeria.

HIV/AIDS in Nigeria

HIV (Human Immunodeficiency Virus) is a virus that weakens the immune system of a person, making them more susceptible to illnesses. It spreads when an infected individual's blood or bodily fluids come into contact with those of an uninfected person. HIV weakens a host's immune system after it has entered the body. As a result, the individual becomes increasingly vulnerable to opportunistic illnesses, which may eventually lead to death. An infected person can take up to a decade to display symptoms, depending on their circumstances and the environment. AIDS (Acquired Immunodeficiency Syndrome) is diagnosed when a person infected with HIV becomes ill as a result of infections.

The first two cases of AIDS in Nigeria were identified in 1985 and reported in 1986 in Lagos, one of whom was a 13-year-old female sex worker from one of West Africa's countries (Nasidi and Harry, 2006). The news of the first AIDS case spread was received with disbelief across the country, because AIDS was thought to be a disease that only affected homosexuals in the United States. Many acronyms arose at the time, one of which was "American Idea for Discouraging Sex", as some individuals interpreted the AIDS tale as a plot by the Americans to discourage sex. However, in 2000, HIV/AIDS was a major concern in Nigeria, with an estimated seven million individuals infected. In 2008, the HIV prevalence rate among individuals aged 15 to 49 was 3.9%; in 2018, the rate was 1.5% among persons aged 15 to 65. The truth is that HIV/AIDS is a global disease that affects millions of people. To take action, the United Nations and other global institutions, governments, regions, organizations, society and individuals must be aware of the problem, its origins, spread, treatment, prevention and other critical issues related to HIV/AIDS, which can be fatal. Five young males in the United States of America were treated with Pneumocystis carinii, a disease that generally affects older persons, between 1980 and 1981. The Centers for Disease Control and Prevention in the United States of America received reports of these incidents and investigated them. As the number of cases grew, scientists realized they were dealing with a distinct sickness. It was given the name AIDS (Ward, 1999).

HIV was discovered to be the cause of AIDS in 1984. The most important data came from a later study conducted in Thailand between 1988 and 1994, which evaluated 200,000 Thais in 1988 and 700,000 Thais in 1994

(Ward, 1999). Scientists can only hypothesize about HIV's origin, although many believe that HIV-2 originated in an African monkey and spread to humans through a sequence of mutations, and that HIV was first carried by African chimpanzees (Kunnuji, 2012). Sexual contact (either heterosexual or homosexual); contact with blood (i.e., blood transfusions or other bodily fluids), blood products or tissues (through needle sharing, i.e., in drug use or poor medical care); accidental needle pricks or breaks in the skin; and transmission from an infected mother to her infant before or during birth and breast-feeding have all been identified as ways for HIV to be transmitted (Dray-Spira, et al., 2012).

In the past, there are no new facts about the virus's transmission, and questions like whether a mosquito that bites a person can spread the virus cannot be answered with assurance. Nigeria has the world's second-largest HIV epidemic and one of the highest new infection rates in Sub-Saharan Africa. Many HIV-positive people in Nigeria are unaware of their condition. Nigeria continues to fall short of the number of HIV testing and counselling locations that are recommended. People living with HIV faced a lack of access to antiretroviral medication, resulting in a high number of AIDS-related deaths in Nigeria. However, the situation is changing. As observed by Dr. Erasmus Morah, the UN AIDS country director in Nigeria,

> the availability of data has expanded to enable the country to truly know its epidemic and its response. Several surveys took place since 2017 which provided precious support to national decision-makers to prioritize, track program performance and mobilize resources to end the epidemic.

The evidence arising from these surveys shows a gradual improvement in HIV treatment since 2017 when the Nigerian government committed to treating 50,000 Nigerians annually (UNAIDS, 2021). This intervention has risen from 55% in 2016 to over 85% in 2020. In 2021, an estimated 90 of people living with HIV (PLHIV) in Nigeria knew their status and most of them have suppressed their viral load (UNAIDS, 2020; 2021).

Types of Media Offerings That Promote Sexuality and HIV/AIDS in Nigeria

Human sexuality would show up constantly in arts and entertainment (Wimmer and Dominick, 2000: 90). One of the major offerings of sexuality in the mass media is pornography. Pornography according to Wimmer and Dominick (2000: 92)

> seems to have become associated with material that features explicit sexual behaviour and nudity in a context frequently characterized by depictions of one character exerting physical or psychological

dominance over one another. Often, this type of material contains explicit violence that is shown and at the same time as explicit sexuality

Glider cited in Hamil (2014) affirms that pornography has grown to the extent it is no longer a taboo; it is the mainstream. Pornography is harmless and mildly enjoyable and is allowed. (Guy, 1985). Ate and Chukwu (2020: 352) gave reasons for the consumption of pornographic materials in Nigeria:

> The first is the marketability and tending nature, the second is the proliferation of online journalism and advertising, the third is the partial adoption of pornographic acts and design by some models. Other factors are lack of strong back-up and gross ethical violation with impunity. . . . Today, pornography is rife in Nigeria due to easy access to it and coupled with the growing appetite of Nigerians on same. The new media structure which is people-driven is a great platform for pornographic products with its high level of reach and access by all and sundry.

Another sexual brand in mainstream and social media is advertising sexual appeals. Five types of sexual information have been identified by Lambiase and Reichert (2003). These are (1) nudity, (2) sexual behaviour, (3) psychical attractiveness, (4) sexual referents and (5) sexual embeds. Nudity is a scenario where a dress by a model is often represented by open blouses with partially exposed cleavages, tight-fitting clothing that highlight the body. In mainstream media nudity is represented by side and back shorts, tub and shower scenes, frontal nudity and waist up. Sexual behaviour is a scenario where models behave sexually in advertising. It can be done through eye contact, inviting smiles, facial expression and sexually provocative steps.

Physical attraction as captured by Lambiase and Reichert (2003) includes displaying the model's alluring physical appearance, facial beauty and complexion and playing a great role in sexual interest. Sexual referents on the other hand involve message elements, visual or verbal, that fertilize sexual thoughts. The last type of sexual information is advertising sexual embeds. The common embeds according to Lambiase and Reichert (2003) are objects that are shaped or positioned like genitalia and small hidden messages, naked people and body parts.

In advertising, the use of women as sexual tools often provokes gender debate among professionals and academics. Adinlewa and Ayara (2019) attest that sexually explicit advertisements have a negative influence on the sexual values of undergraduates of the University of Lagos, Nigeria. Studies also confirm that when consumers do not spend time to reflect on the sexuality of an advertisement, it is possible that may give themselves a chance to focus on other aspects regarding the actual execution of the advertisement (Hedstrom and Harlsson, 2017). The exposure of sexual advertisements on teenagers and youths in may accelerate unprotected sexual intercourse cases which may lead to contracting HIV/AIDs. For instance, home videos are potent mass media tool in the propagation of sexual behaviour in Nigeria. Home video with sexual contents can fuel the desires of teenagers and youth or even adults in having sexual intercourse. Indeed, sexual dance and sexual music videos transmitted through different media platforms can also stimulate careless sexual adventure which may lead to contracting HIV/AIDs. Vanguard (2014) reported on such dances:

> Tiwa Savage and her counterpart, dancehall king, Patoranking have again put up another stunning performance at The Headies awards yesterday after a presentation of Girlie O' remix with so much sensual dances.

The *Punch* (2022) also reported one such scenarios:

> the National Youth Service Corps has faulted corpers seen dancing in a viral video at yet to be identified orientation camp. In a video, one female corper was seen giving a lap dance to a male counterpart . . . A male corper was seen hitting his organ against the female own, with a corper heard saying, "give am well".

It is important to stress that both the social media and mainstream media have reported this sexually alluring dance to millions of Nigerians. The effect of that on the youth could be counterproductive viewed from a sexuality perspective. While it is observed that sexual contents in Nigerian movies are perceived as bad by the audience (Uwom, Chioma, and Sodeinde, 2013), it is clearly held that risky sexual behaviour triggered by the media can be instrumental to the spread of HIV/AIDS (Rokhmah and Khorion, 2015). It is against this backdrop that UNAIDS (2004) believes that media organizations have an enormous influence in education and empowering individuals to avoid contracting HIV/AIDS.

Conclusion

The study reveals that pornography is a major theme in the media on sexuality. It shows that social media and the internet are the leading media of sexuality in Nigeria. This finding has questioned the agenda setting power of the mass media which has been dwindled as a result of the breakdown of the gatekeeping concept of the media. It revealed that sexuality media has led some media audience to risky sexual behaviour that nose-dive into contracting HIV/AIDS. It concludes that different media offerings topped by pornography promote sexuality and by extension contraction of HIV/AIDS in Nigeria. Hence, policy action on the accessibility of online media contents is a vital intervention to address the social determinant of HIV/AIDS in Nigeria.

References

Adinlewa, T. and Ayara, M.G. (2019) Influence of Sexually Explicit Advertisements on the Sexual Values of Undergraduates of University of Lagos, Nigeria. *Novena Journal of Communication*, 9: 58–69.

Amanze, C.U. (2006). The Socio-economic Impact of AIDS Scourge in Developing Countries. In Daura, M.M. (Ed.), *Nigeria's Technical Aid Corps: Issues and Perspectives*. Ibadan: Dokun Publishing House.

Asekun-Olarinmoye, O.S., Asekun-Olarinmoye, E.O., Adebimpe, W.O., and Omisore, A.G. (2014). Effects of Mass Media and Internet on Sexual Behaviour of Undergraduates in Osogbo Metropolis, South Western Nigeria. *Adolescence Health Medicine Therapeutics*, 5: 15–23. http://dx.doi.org/10.2147/AHMT.S54339.

Ate, A.A. (2008). *Media and Society*. Lagos: National Open University of Nigeria.

Ate, A.A. and Chukwu, O.J. (2020). Hunting the Beat of Pornography of Pornography in Nigeria: Theoretical, Legal and Ethical Perspectives. *Confluence Law Journal*, 6(2), 207–215.

Ate, A.A. (n.d.). *Theories of Mass Communication*. Ikeji-Arakeji: Joseph Ayo Babalola University Publishing.

Ate, A.A. and Ikerodah, J.O. (2019). Mass Communication Students Perception of Fake News Phenomenon in Nigeria. *Journal of Media, Communication and Languages*, 6(1): 131–141.

Brown, J.D. (2002). Mass Media Influence on sexuality. *Journal of Sex Research*, 39(1): 221–230.

Davis, D.K. and Robinson, J.P. (1989). Newsflow and Democratic Society. In Constock, G. (Ed.), *Public Communication and Behaviour* (Vol. 2). Orlando, FA: Academic Press.

Dennis, E.E. (1991). The Media Are Quite Powerful. In Dennis, E.E. and Merrikl, J.C. (Eds.), *Media Debates: Issues in Mass Communication*. London: Longman Publishing Group.

Dray-Spira, R., Legeai, C., Le Den, M., Boué, F., LascouxCombe, C., Simon, A., and Meyer, L. (2012). Burden of HIV disease and comorbidities on the chances of maintaining employment in the era of sustained combined antiretoviral therapies use. *AIDS*, 26(2), 207–215.

European Expert Group on Sexuality Education. (2015). Sexuality Education – What Is It? *Sexuality, Society and Learning*, 16(4): 427–431.

Garlick, S. (2011). A new sexual Revolution? *Critical Theorry/Pornography and the Internet, Canadian Review of Sociology*, 48(2) 221–239.

Griffin, E.M. (2000). *A First Look at Communication Theory*. Boston: McGraw Hill.

Griffin, E.M. (2012). *A First Look at Communication Theory* (8th ed.). New York: McGraw Hill.

Gruber, E. and Grube, J.W. (2000). Adolescent, Sexuality and the Media. *Western Journal of Medicine*, 172(3): 210–214. http://dx.doi.org/10.1136/ewjm.172.3.210.

Guy, D. (1985). Notes Towards a Theory of Pornography. *Sun Magazine*. https://www.thesunmagazine.org/issues/115/notes-toward-a-theory-of-pornography. Accessed 15 February 2023.

Hamil, J. (2014) Porn Brand Behind 21st Century Playboy's Plans. A Hardcare Future for Journalism. *Forbes*, 16 May. https://www.forbes.com/sites/jasperhamill/2014/05/16/porn-brand-behind-21st-century-playboy-plans-a-hardcore-future-for-journalism/?sh=29f75b4a5567. Accessed 15 February 2023.

Harris, P. (1989). *A Cognitive Psychology of Mass Communication*. Hilldale, NJ: Lawrence Erlbaum Associates.

Hedstrom, J. and Harlsson, J. (2017). Consumers' Attitudes Toward Sexual Appeal in Advertising. A project submitted to Lulea University of Technology, Department of

Business Administration, Technology and Social Sciences. https://www.diva-portal.org/smash/get/diva2:1114476/FULLTEXT01.pdf.

Katz, D. (1959). A functional approach to the study of attitudes. *Public Opinion Quarterly*, 24(2), 163–204.

Kunnuji, M. (2012). Online Sexual Activities and Sexual Risk-taking among Adolescents and Young Adults in Lagos Metropolis, Nigeria. *African Journal of Reproductive Health*, 16(2): 207–218.

Lambiase, J. and Reichert, T. (2003). *Sex in Advertising*. Mahwah, NJ: Lawrence Erlbaum Associates.

McQuail, D. (2000). *Mass Communication* (4th ed.). London: Sage Publication.

Murphy, D.R. (1997). *Mass Communication and Human Interactions*. Boston, MA: Houston Mifflin Company.

Nasidi, A., and Harry, T. O. (2006). "The epidemiology of HIV/AIDS in Nigeria". In Adeyi, O. Kanki, P. J., Odutolu, O. and Idoko, J.A. (Eds.), *AIDS in Nigeria: A Nation on the Threshold*. Massachusetts: Harvard University Press.

Nworgu, K.O. (2020). Mass Media and Premarital Sexual Behaviour of the Adolescents in Imo State Nigeria. *Edições Anteriores*, 7(17): 1257–1270.

Oladele, T.T., Olakunde, B.O., Oladele, A.O., Ugbuoyi, S., and Yamey, G. (2020). The Impact of COVID 19 on HIV Financing in Nigeria: A Call for Proactive Measure. *BMJ Glob Health*, 5(5): e002718. http://dx.doi.org/10.1136/bmjgh-2020-002718.

Punch. (2022, 16 March). Viral Video: NYSC Reacts to Corpers' Erotic Dance at Orientation Camp. https://punchng.com/viral-video-nysc-reacts-to-corpers-erotic-dance-at-orientation-camp/.

Rokhmah, D. and Khorion, P. (2015). The Role of Textual Behaviour in the Transmission of HIV/AIDS in Adolescent in Coastal Area. *Procedia Environmental Sciences*, 23: 99–104.

UNAIDS. (2004). The Media & HIV/AIDS: Making the Difference. https://data.unaids.org/publications/irc-pub06/jc1000-media_en.pdf.

UNAIDS. (2019). "Global Update 2019 – Communities at the Centre". Available at https://www.unaids.org/en/resources/documents/2019/2019-global-AIDS-update

UNAIDS. (2020). Global HIV & AIDS Statistics-Fact Sheet. https://www.unaids.org/en/resources/fact-sheet.

UNAIDS. (2021). "Five questions about the HIV response in Nigeria". Retrieved 27 August 2022 from https://www.unaids.org/en/resources/presscentre/featurestories/2021/october/five-questions-nigeria

UNESCO. (2018). International Technical Guidance on Sexuality Education. https://www.unfpa.org/sites/default/files/pub-pdf/ITGSE.pdf.

Uwom, O.O., Chioma, P.E., and Sodeinde, O.A. (2013). Audience Perception of Sexual Contents in Nigeria Movies. *New Media and Mass Communication*, 19: 16–24.

Vanguard. (2014, 15 December). Again, Tiwa, Patoranking Thrill Audience with Sensual Dance. https://allafrica.com/stories/201412152192.html.

Ward, L.M., Erickson, S.E., Lippman, J.R., and Giaccardi, S. (2016). Sexual Media Content and Effects. *Oxford Research Encyclopedias*. https://oxfordre.com/communication/display/10.1093/acrefore/9780190228613.001.0001/acrefore-9780190228613-e-2;jsessionid=0478B1E29A79302E17CC69D7A286FDD4?rskey=75ihDR&result=9.

World Health Organization (WHO). (2006). Defining Sexual Health. https://www.who.int/teams/sexual-and-reproductive-health-and-research/key-areas-of-work/sexual-health/defining-sexual-health.

Wimmer, R.D. and Dominick, J.R. (2000). *Mass Media Research: An Introduction*. London: Walsworth Publishing Company.

Part IV

Socio-Political Determinants of Illness and Wellness in the African Literary Discourse

9 Traditional Medicine and Public Health in Postcolonial African Literary Discourse

Ngetcham and Njouonap Gbetnkom Assiatou

Introduction

Before the advent of Western medicine, African forbearers depended largely on traditional medicine for the treatment of ailments and cure of various types of diseases. Traditional medicine is defined as the "belief and experiences indigenous to different cultures, used in the maintenance of health as well as in the prevention, diagnosis, improvement or treatment of physical and mental illnesses" (Orgah and Orgah, 2015: 2). Africans believe that the cause of ill health, misfortunes, and other afflictions could be traced to both the visible and the invisible elements of the world. Since most people do not have the ability to communicate with the forces that controlled healing and well-being in the world, the medicine men became very useful (Magesa, 1997: 210). A traditional healer is one who provides medical care in the community where he lives, using herbs, minerals, animal parts, incantations, and other methods, based on the cultures and beliefs of his people. Traditional healers are of four different types: diviners, herbalists, traditional birth attendants, and bone setters (Faleye and Akande, 2019). They act as the link between the people and the supernatural realm, and so people consult them frequently (Magesa, 1997: 209–212).

This chapter investigates the role of African medicine men healers and the impact of modern medicine in postcolonial African societies. Orthodox medicine has, to a very large extent, been useful in disease control. Nevertheless, modern medicine has mainly succeeded in dealing with the physical aspects of ill-health (Mumo, 2012: 112). Ngetcham in the archaeological approach of literary texts sees a literary text as a "terrain, site, champ de fouille, de repérage des débris, d'enquêtedans des ruine, de collecte de resteou de vestige" (English translation; field, a site, field of excavation, of debris discovery, investigations on ruins, to collect the rest of vestiges) (Ngetcham, 2022: 34). Using this approach permits the reconstruction of real society through fictive characters and events. It takes a literary text not only as a document but also as a field of potential vestiges or real world in the writing universe. It is a visible manifestation of values integrated by the community of its author and therefore becomes a reference of values transmitted from

DOI: 10.4324/9781003429135-14

generation to generation. From this method of reading literary works, traces of herbal, ritual, and spiritual aspects of African healing will be identified. Taking as corpus some postcolonial novels – *Seat of Thorns* by Francis Ateh (2018), *Verdict of the Gods* by Janet Ekaney (2007), *Burning Grass* Cyprian by Ekwensi (1962), and *Efuru* by Flora Nwapa (1966) – this chapter identifies traces through which the holistic healing of the African peoples is portrayed and the traces that mark the presence of the modern healing methods.

Added to this approach, due to the evolution the world is witnessing nowadays, the postcolonial theory of Eduard Glissant in *Poetics of Relation* is deployed to establish cordial attitudes towards Western treatment. Here, Glissant opposes the "notion of being rooted" (1997: 11) that aims to "break the social bond", prompting the knowledge that identity is no longer completely within the root but also in relation with the other. Therefore, this theory will determine one of the full senses of the postcolonial era which is provided by the actions of human cultures identifying one another for their mutual interaction as far as assuring people's health is concerned.

The African Holistic Healing in Postcolonial Literature

African medical culture addresses physical, biological, environmental and spiritual aspects of societal wellbeing (Mumo, 2012; Faleye and Akande, 2019). In the context of African medicinal inheritance, the vast majority have some knowledge of traditional medicine which is often inherited and passed down through the generations through folklore. This means that a medicine man would pass on the profession to his children or other younger relatives. After Elome II has shown to his son Ngole some roots for the cure of certain ailments, he tells the latter: "My father showed it to me just as I am showing you" (*VOG*, 16). About Sango Abwe who heals barrenness, it is narrated, "his ability to help barren women was said to have been handed down to him by his late grand father" (*VOG*, 63). In Efuru, the *dibia* tells his patients: "I inherited all my medicines from my father, who inherited them from his father" (*Efuru*, 34). Equally, when Elome II asks what to pay the diviner after consultation and asked what to pay him, the latter replies: "Pay me? . . . nothing, . . . my grand father handed down this knowledge to me free of charge. How can I ask people to pay me for it? He would probably turn in his grave if I did that. I am happy if I can help anyone" (*VOG*, 103). Because secrecy and competition surround the use of traditional medications, the healers are therefore reluctant to hand their knowledge to anyone but trusted relatives. They stay firm to the rules transferred to them by their forefathers, if not they will find the medicine losing its efficacy. As a result, the payment of the majority of these medicine men is the satisfaction they derive from helping others solve their problems.

Healing through the traditional view lays no interest in money making, because the solidarity among Africans does not only stop at the level of sharing ordinary material but also at assuring weaker people's well-being. This is why whenever a medicine man takes a reward after healing a patient, it is usually symbolic than for money making. The respect of this helps in the preservation and conservation of the ancestral healing methods. Their aim is therefore to protect and serve the interest of members of their communities who use their services. To prove this, Liverpool notes, "Traditional healers are accessible options for people with limited financial resources" (Liverpool, 2004: 825). The continuum of indigenous medical practices of herbalism, divination, ancestral sacrifice, spiritual exorcism, and midwifery illustrates this reality in postcolonial Africa.

Herbalism

Herbal medicine is a special and prominent form of traditional medicine in which the traditional healer specializes in the use of herbs to treat various ailments. Its administration is through a good knowledge of herbs and roots and the right application to the patients who need them (Ekeopara and Azubuike: 39). In *Burning Grass* (*BG* henceforth), Sunsaye is a "great medicine-man", who, when his son is sick, "He took a decoction of roots and herbs to Rikku and sat beside him. . . . It was warm and throbbing" (*BG*, 7–8). These decoctions are made by boiling woody pieces for a specified period of time and filtering. The medicine men make the decoction mostly with dried herbs and fresh ones sometimes. The herbs can be ground, sliced for better infusion. It produces antibodies that combat various diseases. Medicine men are also consulted to treat barrenness. After their marriage, Ahone and Elome II have difficulties conceiving. Ahone meets the first herbalist where "[s]he was . . . given a concoction to take home. . . . Ahone continued the treatment for six months . . ." (62). When this did not work, the couple turned to another native doctor known as Sango Abwe. Sango Abwe noted that "he would stop the treatment if the new medicine is ineffective" (63).

His precision on the period for which the medicine has to be taken is due to the fact that every prescription according to the nature of the illness has specific instructions on the dose and the time frame. The medicine man speaks the truth to Ahone because, for him to be respected and more valued, he needs to be competent and most of all a trusted agent to his patients. Herbs are equally used to interrupt poison. On a trek with his son Ngole, Elome II passes over to him a medicine against poison as quoted:

Do you see that creeping grass near that big tree? . . . that red one . . . My son, that grass works wonders. It neutralises the effect of poison, instantly. If you suspect that someone has been poisoned, simply give him the leaf to chew and that will do it.

(*VOG*, 15)

Medicines against poison are mostly used for both curative and preventive methods. About his father from whom he learns a great deal of these medicines, he says,

> When I was much younger than you, I remember that he took care of our little ailments himself, like headache, stomach-ache, convulsion and so on. He would simply go behind his house, pick a leaf, give any of us who had a particular ailment to chew and that would be it.
>
> (16)

The ease with which traditional medicine is made is due to what Ekeopara and Azubuike note as "its cultural acceptability, affordability, and accessibility" (2017: 32). In this regard, one sees that, apart from the medicine men, every parent in his household has specific traditional treatment they offer their children.

In *Efuru*, many of these instances are identified where mothers offer traditional treatments to their children for convulsion. Convulsion in a child is caused by fever and is the most serious symptom which occurs in childhood. Ajanupu narrates about his son:

> He had convulsion yesterday. . . . One day he felt unwell so I gave him some tablets I got for the dispensary. Then just as I was about to leave. . . . I hear a shout. . . . It was Nnoro, he was having a convulsion. . . . Then I took kernel oil and emptied the whole contents on his body, head and face. Then I mixed some with mentholetum and put it in his anus. . . . It was much better after that. I gave him some purgative medicine and today he was playing with the children outside.
>
> (*Efuru*, 16)

The failure of the tablets to cure the child shows that a number of traditional medicines are important and effective therapeutic regimens in the management of a wide spectrum of diseases some of which may not be effectively managed using orthodox medicines. According to Abdullahi (2011: 117), traditional medicine "is thought to be desirable and necessary for treating a range of health problems that medical science does not treat adequately". Kernel oil is used in calming down the nerves of convulsing children. It can be used singly or mixed with menthol to ease the children to pass out something. When Efuru's daughter convulses and she gives her the same treatment, the child feels better but later develops fever again: "Ajanupu then rubbed more kernel oil on her this time mixed with some leaves", and, she says, "That's all I know. . . . This is all I give to my children when they have fever to prevent them from having convulsion" (65). Used alone or mixed with leaves, kernel oil serves as both curative and preventive methods for convulsion. It is notable that the healing was achieved using natural materials from the environment without recourse to the payment of hospital bills or the use of any invasive procedure of medical science. The different steps of the treatment are followed by purgating the child who needs his organ cleaned. Purgative medicine is prepared with herbs and other mixtures. Gilbert's mother tells:

> My stomach is dirty. So I took some purgative medicines. . . . You pick the leaves and use it in cooking some nice yam pottage. Then eat it first thing in the morning. . . . I feel clean inside. It is the purgative medicine I give my children when their stomachs are dirty.
>
> (138–139)

Purgation is effective in cleaning the digestive system of individuals of different age groups and avoiding convulsions in children.

When Sunsaye is sick in *BG*, "Rikku and Shaitu, with the aid of all the herbs they knew, doctored him" (118). The role of herbal treatment is very remarkable since it arises from a thorough knowledge of the medicinal properties of indigenous plants. These first treatments are general care services; "they are health services provided to patients by non-specialised health care providers" (Ekeopara and Azubuike, 38). The general care services regularly work because the non-specialized healthcare providers have not gotten their knowledge of the herbs from a vacuum but it is indigenous knowledge gotten from their people who have been using the medicines before. In traditional societies, therefore, people do not hesitate to give the first treatment to their sick family members with no fear of risk, and they can only meet a medicine man when the state of the person has not gotten positive results. Herbal medicine is freely available and can easily be accessed by all.

Divination and Sacrifice to the Ancestors

Divination means consulting the spirit world to acquire wellness. Because of the revealing powers of divination, it is usually the first step in African traditional treatment.

As a result, no treatment is efficient so far as the cause of the poor health is not diagnosed. In *VOG*, when Elome II snatches the young girl his uncle of more than 60 years wants to spend his last days on earth with, the latter "secretly went to consult his oracles" (*VOG*,54–56) and inflicts the couple with barrenness. This proves that one can inflict sickness on his enemy through the invocation of curses in the name of the ancestors and the gods. After two years of consultation with herbalists, there is no result.

This is because the couple relies firstly on the physical aspect by first going to herbalists rather than the spiritual. When the condition of the patient is not improved after the application of simple treatments, the method of divination is applied. The patient meets the diviner for spiritual guidance and recommendation of the type of medicine to be applied for a quick cure. After the seventh year of marriage with the two wives, he decides with the elders to consult a diviner. Sango Sube, the one responsible for the illness, is chosen to meet a diviner, but after consultation, he hides the real cause and reveals the ancestors are angry against Elome II because "he hadn't make sacrifices to them since he became the Paramount Chief. So, the medicine man advised that sacrifices be made to appease the gods and brings blessings to Elome II and the family" (85). Some treatment may involve ritual practices such as animal sacrifices to appease the gods when the ailment is envisaged to be caused by the afflictions of the gods.

The delay makes Elome II and one of his uncles to start doubting the honesty of Sango Sube and they decide to meet other diviners. Sango Etape first goes to a diviner who uses a "white, medium-size life cock with its feet strapped together" (93) to find out his clients' ailments. The cock's reaction determines its reply. It is asked if the barrenness is caused by Elome II, his wives or their families, or ancestors, and "the cock made no sign" (94). When it is asked whether it is from any member of Elome's family, "Hardly had the medicine man completed the sentence when the cock moves its head forward and backwards" (94). It later reveals it is a man. When Elome II hears this, he decides to go and verify from another medicine man, who in turn uses "a wooden bowl and the tooth of a tiger . . . placed the tooth in the bowl and filled it with water" for divination. He equally asks the first group of questions like the medicine man Sango Atape meets; "there was still no reaction" (100). When asked if it is from Elome II's family members, "The tooth of the tiger started rising slowly to the surface with little bubbles forming around it. Slowly again, it sank to the bottom of the bowl" (101). It later on reveals the person is a man and adds in his turn that it is an old man. Medicine men take their time to find out the root cause of a problem and decide on the line of action to take. This goes in line with Mumo's belief about traditional healers that "they also detected witches, sorcerers and other evil persons and forces that hindered productivity" (Mumo, 2012: 116). When the culprit does not come up to reveal his deeds, the medicine man later prescribes the treatment:

> Take this powder. When you return to your village, on the third day of your return, get up at first cockcrow and sprinkle the powder round your house. If you return to bed, never open the door before midmorning even if somebody came to wake you up, or even if you heard cries in another compound. Do that, and upon your return, the person would tell you his name.
>
> (106)

When Elome II does as told, the following morning, Sango Sube dies after sudden illness. The medicine man they call to heal him refuses because "he accused him of violating somebody's compound" (109). Some days later after his death, Elome II marries a third wife and "within a short time, the girl was pregnant" (110). The diviners strive to discover the root causes of illness and how to prevent them from recurring. This medicine man's aims have been therefore to diagnose, treat and prevent the barrenness following his expertise in divination. The end result is the sad end of the chief's uncle. The prescription of the powder and its effectiveness abides with the African people mentality that "the religious specialists neutralized the evil and suffering brought by witches, wizards and other evil forces" (Mumo, 115).

In *Efuru*, when Efuru and her husband have difficulty conceiving, her father tells her, "Something must be done, my daughter. It is not in our blood. Our women are productive. There must be a reason for this. We shall see a *dibia*" (*Efuru*, 24). This statement implies the age-old knowledge of genetics in African medical practice. Added to the belief that a disease can be an affliction from the gods, ancestors or people, it can equally be inherited. So, since their ancestors were productive, the future generation is likely to be. On their arrival, the dibia breaks kola nut for welcoming his guests and divination: "The *dibia* took the kola nut and broke it. There were only three pieces. He looked at it closely and shook his head" (26). In African tradition, Kola nut serves as a medium of communication between God and man. The number of pieces is the maximum number of children she can have. The dibia reveals after breakage: "Your daughter is not barren. She will have a baby next year if she will only do what I am going to ask her to do. Again she has not got many children . . . She will sacrifice to the ancestors . . . Next year during the Owu festival if nothing happens to you, come back to me" (*Efuru*, 26). He speaks of Efuru's situation when he is not told. It seems obvious that the dibia has an intuitive capacity to gain insight into the client's and life situation. The sacrifice is to appease the gods, if ever, she has violated any community rule. So done as said, Efuru, after some months, falls pregnant and put to birth a baby girl. Special concoctions are prepared to clean the reproductive organs of barren women, while rituals can accompany such administration if it is believed that there is a spiritual agency involved in the barrenness. When she and her husband go to thank the dibia with some gifts and again:

> He broke the kola nut, and frowned with pain. "Our fathers forbid, God forbid. God won't agree this. . . . We have only two pieces of kola. It is not a good sign my children. Njeri, bring another kola." . . . The dibia broke. Again, there were only two pieces. "This is strange my children. My children come again on Eke day". . . . "Something will be wrong. I can prevent it. But I must be given time. I have seen it, but not clearly yet. Our fathers will help me. I shall sacrifice to them. I shall ask their aid." The dibia said slowly to himself. . . . On Nkwo day, a day to the appointed day, Efuru heard that the dibia was dead. He died in his sleep.
> (35)

The little the number of the pieces, the higher the rate of misfortune it implies. Two pieces of kola highly determine death or any misfortune. The double breakage too, of the kola and the acquisition of the same result, is a clear indication that there is no prevention. The divination being reserved for Efuru's family, she does not have the chance to be revealed. So, her ignorance about what the dibia has seen finally makes the bad event to happen. When her daughter falls sick,

> it was only then that she remembered what the dibia told her and Adizua when they went to him after the birth of Ogonim. The dibia after breaking the kola nut saw that something was wrong. He was not sure what it was, "What did he see?" Efuru asked herself. . . . She was very frightened.
>
> (66)

With their ability to deal with the unseen, and the supernatural, these dibias are held in high esteem in the community, because they are believed to have extra-sensory perception and can see beyond the ordinary man. To this effect, what he might have seen may have to do with her daughter. After some days of illness, Ogonim dies. Therefore, the medicine men are the eyes of the people; they equally act at preventing certain catastrophes to happen in the lives of the people.

When Adizua's mother is sick and a diviner is called, he reveals after consultation,

> It is the absence of her only son that makes her ill. . . . I will not give her medicine. No medicine will cure her. She will have to sacrifice to the ancestors and to the gods, so that they will turn the heart of her son towards home.
>
> (*Efuru*, 158)

When she hears of the possibility of seeing her son one day, her mood changes, and then "[t]he sacrifice was performed and she felt better" (159). As an intermediary between the visible and the invisible worlds, the diviner here determines which spirit is at work and what Adizua's mother can do to be healed, and her son's heart will turn back home and get into harmony with the ancestors. This is a psychological health intervention through divination and sacrifice in African traditional medicine. This form of holistic medicine is alien to medical science.

About Adizua's father who equally abandons his wife, he comes back one day and as narrated by his wife,

> This time he was very ill. He had contracted a bad disease and had come to me to heal him. I took him to a dibia. The dibia said he had annoyed the ancestors and have to receive his punishment. . . . I went to the market on Nkwo day to buy the things the dibia had asked me to buy and before I came back, Adizua's father was dead.
>
> (61)

When an individual annoys the gods, it suggests there has been a violation of an established order from the side of the sick man. These established norms are taboos and traditional healers are of the opinion that disobeying taboos is one of the ways that could lead to severe illness to the person involved. This is because these taboos form an important part of African traditional religion and cultural norms. These are things, or a way of life, that are forbidden by a community.

The belief and trust in diviners is also identified in *Seat of Thorns (SOT* henceforth). When Ndong reaches Ningang and decides to indigenize Christianity, this means "loss of influence, popularity and poverty" for his Catechist and the latter starts planning evil against the young priest. Ndong's cousin reveals to him: "I want to give you some information from Kaleiti, the big medicine man. . . . He has asked you to be careful with the Catechist who may be planning some evil against you" (*SOT*, 41). Ndong doubts his cousin but the latter who is a pure traditionalist reminds him: "One never knows. But you know Kaleiti is a great seer who would not joke with something like that. I suggest you watch the Catechist closely" (Id). According to Ndong and his Christian beliefs, God would not allow any harm to befall him. His resistance to believe according to Mumo's point of view is because "the Bible teaches that behind genuinely extra ordinary supernatural Powers of African Traditional Religions is the work of demonic spirits. . . . God forbids any involvement whatsoever with mystical powers of any sort whether they are socially acceptable or anti-social" (Mumo, 114). When he is informed about the petitions, the Catechist has sent to the Bishop about his practices in the village, "Ndong resolved to watch the Catechist more closely: "Did Kaleiti not send Bong to warn him about the Catechist?" (69). This petition leads to his dismissal from the Catholic Mission. Thus, the neglect of divination can cause considerable devastation in people's life. According to Swantz, a medicine man is considered as a strong and powerful man of the spirit, for his ability rests not only in his medicine but in his Baraka, a word which means blessings but is often used in this sense as the medicine man's gift of inner power" (Swantz, 1990: 25). This justifies why Kaleiti is looked upon with respect, if not with a little awe and wonder, because of his ability to divine and to know the secret things in life.

Spirituality and Exorcism

Many of the traditional communities' belief has a mental set that illness, especially mental illness, is mostly caused by evil spirits. Power is one of the fundamental objects that people will do all to acquire, even if it means ruining the life of the other. When Sunsaye is in power, he has a rival named Ardo, who inflicts Sunsaye with the *sokugo*: "that charm of the Fulani cattlemen; a magic that turned studious men into wanderers, that led husbands to desert their wives, Chiefs their people and sane men their reason" (10). The enemy inflicts this mental illness by sending a dove: "A talisman – a small rectangular white fold of parchment – was clearly visible to Sunsaye. It trailed after the dove as it skipped. With his weak eyes he followed the bird's movement" (9). When the victim sees this dove, he follows and "felt he could easily grow wings and overtake the dove" (10). In the Fulani communities in West Africa, "A man could send his enemy wandering to his death by striking him with the *sokugo*, the wondering charm" (12). The Ardo successfully scatters Sunsaye's family and takes over. In this regard, only one who has metaphysical power can heal him.

On his wandering around, he goes to the homes of his sons: Jalla and Hodio. He equally visits Ligu's camp and other places. Though all of them suspect he is charmed, he convinces them that he is looking for his son's lover, Fatimeh. If no one removes the charm, the victim can vanish, never to come back again. When he finds Fatimeh, she finds out that all the excuses for bringing her home to marry Rikku are not voluntary. She realizes this when she is with him and has no plan to leave, he suddenly breaks to leave after seeing a "dove, flying south". After holding him back, she exclaims, "Your eyes are all red, your tongue is out. Father, you have the wandering sickness" (102). The colour of his eyes and the position of his tongue are signs to identify this illness. With this remark, having learnt a great deal about herbs, she sets up to free Sunsaye from the charm:

> She began to mix some powders on a wooden slab, and presently she brought out some cold milk and stirred it in. The powders made the milk look green. All the while, she talked. Then she lifted the bowls and said: "drink this: drink it, and whoever it is that made that medicine – that's right! From now on the sokugo departs from your body. Your body is rid forever of the spirit." She began to mutter words and soon she fell into a trance while Mai Sunsaye made a weary face at the taste of the mixture.
>
> (102–103)

The uttering of words and falling in trance is to exorcise the spirits taking control of the patient's soul. These uttering of words are psychologically vital, and they play a great role in the healing of the sick person. Together with herbs, she successfully heals Sunsaye through exorcism. The mixture of the herb and the powder accompanied with the trance portrays the physical and spiritual nature of the illness. Even though Sunsaye looks physically well, Fatimeh finds out about his psychological problem. This proves that his treatment does not only involve aiding his physical being but also involves the spiritual, moral, and social components of being as well, since after this infliction, he fails in some moral and numerous social aspects of his life. First of all as a husband or father, as chief and likewise, a medicine man is expected to heal patients instead of wandering around. Exorcism is hence performed for those who are mentally challenged. In this view, until the possessed person is delivered from the power of the evil spirit, the person will not gain his freedom.

Midwifery Services in Traditional Communities

Midwifery is a healthcare profession in which providers give prenatal care to expecting mothers, attend to the birth of their infants, and provide post-partum care to the mother and her infant. A midwife is a person who assists the mother at childbirth and who initially acquired her skills delivering babies by herself or by working with other birth attendants (Ekeopara and Azubuike, 2017: 35). In postcolonial Africa, rural-urban inequality has led to the concentration of orthodox medical services in the urban centres. Consequently, the poor reach of orthodox medical service means that many inhabitants of the rural areas must continue to rely on traditional birth attendants for child delivery. The following extracts show how traditional midwives intervene during childbirth in rural communities in postcolonial Africa:

> Her labour started at first cockcrow. By late morning, she was still in serious pains. Lucy Etane could bear it no longer. She sent somebody to Esele village to get a renowned traditional midwife. When the midwife saw the patient, she smiled and joked that the child wanted to know its father before it came out. . . . "If you tell us the name of the father of the child it will come out" . . . "Elome II!" the girl yelled . . . Elome II! Messang, yelled again, and at once, the child was born.
>
> (*VOG*, 110)

> That night Efuru did not sleep. She tossed in bed. She woke her mother-in-law. . . . The old woman went to call her sister. . . . Ajanupu came with her immediately. . . . "Lie down" she commanded Efuru. . . . "That's the head. . . . Now you are to do exactly as I say. If you are afraid, you will have a weak and sickly baby. If you do exactly as I tell you, you will have a strong and healthy baby. . . ." Efuru did as she was told. In about half an hour she delivered her baby. . . . Single handed, Ajanupu attended to both mother and child. . . . It was easy for her. . . . She had eight children. It was only the first and second that she was helped to deliver. All the others she delivered herself.
>
> (*Efuru*, 31)

As shown in these extracts, people patronize traditional midwifery for their maternal and post-partum health problems. In the first extract, it is seen how they can handle delivery cases intelligibly. They have tact and methods to make women whose delivery is complicated to give birth. Through their methods, it is seen they are specialists in low-risk pregnancy, childbirth, and post-partum care. They help women to have healthy pregnancy and natural birth experience. For neonatal treatment, the midwives follow up pregnant women till their birth and after birth. This is seen in *Efuru* when she is pregnant and when Ajanupu comes to their house and she and her mother-in-law are eating Ogbono soup:

> "Ossai . . . Don't you know that ogbono soup is not good for an expected mother? . . . Okra is not good. Snail is not good also. If she eats snails her baby will have plenty of saliva" . . . she listed all the don't's of a pregnant woman. She was not to go out at night. . . . When she is sitting down, nobody must cross her leg. . . . At the seven month, Efuru noticed that her legs were swollen. . . . She told her mother-in-law who imme-diately told her sister. . . . The next day, she brought some leaves and some palm wine. She cooked the leaves adding a little palm wine. . . . She gave some to Efuru to drink . . . "every morning and night, you warm it over a slow fire, put some palm wine in it and drink" . . . Efuru kept to the instructions religiously. The medicine worked. She discovered that she urinated more and that her legs and feet were no longer swollen. She had no trouble after that.
>
> (*Efuru*, 28–29)

The pregnant women go through counselling. That is, they are counselled on the dos and don'ts of their state of health. When she puts to bed and after five months, Ajanupu advices they should put alligator pepper in the child's mouth to free her tongue; if not, "the baby might be deaf and dumb" (33). Again, when Efuru complains her breasts are dried to breastfeed the child, Ajanupu advices her " 'to drink plenty of palm wine, meanwhile I am going to treat you'. She chewed some palm kernels which she used in rub-bing her breasts. 'This will help,' . . . Efuru was all right. Her breasts was full . . .' " (33). In the traditional healing system, midwives therefore prepare these women physically and mentally for pregnancy, childbirth, and the post-partum stage.

Modern Medicine in Traditional Societies

Orthodox medicine has succeeded in dealing with the physical aspects of ill-health. Even though the African medicine men continue with their trade in spite of the changes that have taken place in the continent, "many Afri-cans also combine modern drugs with traditional medicines" (Mumo, 2009: 73), though some develop phobic mentalities for the latter. *In Efuru*, when Nwozuis is ill, his wife nurses him: "she went to a dibia who gave her some leaves to boil for her husband" (*Efuru*, 95), but, the situation worsens. They decide to see a doctor. When his problem is diagnosed, he is given an injec-tion but told he will have to go through a surgery in the hospital because his illness has "something to do with the male organ" (97). Nwabata, his wife, is against the operation as she opines, "I don't trust these Doctors . . . They'll first 'kill' you, then do the operation, and after, if they know they cannot cure you, they give you poison" (98). Her reaction portrays her phobic mindsets towards this treatment and, thus, the fear of the other. Her behaviour is also justified by the mental setting that herbal treatment is considered in this community to be a lot safer than orthodox medicine, being natural in origin.

At last, Nwozu is finally operated and "the operation was successful and Nwosu remained there for a fort-night. By the time he came back, he was a changed man. He looked fresh and healthier" (102). The success of the treatment surprises his wife such that she approves, "So there is so much life in you, my husband. These white people are great, they are deep" (102). When it comes to illnesses that necessitate surgery, Western treatment is highly recommended. When Nnona has problems with her legs and meets the doctor, after examination, he says, ". . . 'it will take a long time to heal'. . . . She had a bad sore and she allowed it to eat into the bones. I shall send her to the hospital where she will have an operation" (130). After the operation, "she spent two months in the hospital and Nnona came home cured . . . She was looking very fit" (130).

Equally, when Efuru falls ill, "many dibias were contacted and all of them gave different diagnosis; some said she was going to have a baby, others said the gods were angry with her . . ." (215). With all these dibias contacted, different treatments are prescribed like, especially, the sacrifice for the ancestors' appeasement. When it is said "she is guilty of adultery" and must confess before she gets well, knowing that the revelation is false, she abandons the possibility to be healed by the traditional treatment. This incoherence among the medicine men portrays that in certain cases of illnesses, Western medicine is important. In this regard, she argues, "Ajanupu saved me. . . . She took me to the hospital in Aba. I was cured. I came back only a month ago" (220). This portrays that the traditional treatment is not always effective in most of the physical aspects, and thus, there is need for modern treatment intervention. Therefore, with the coming of orthodox medicine, they consult modern doctors when they have not achieved desired results from the traditional treatment.

Some people believe that injections are more effective in curing illnesses than taking drugs. In a passage, Gilbert mother's friend tells her after she has been to a doctor, "You know I have been suffering from "bad blood". So I went to the doctor and had an injection. I am feeling much better now" (181). When she tells her friend she will also go to a doctor who will give her injections, her friend asks her to wait for Efuru, she opposes, "No, I won't wait for Efuru. She will take me to Doctor Uzaru who never gives injections" (181). From their mental setting perspective, these women are of the opinion that "No cure is effective without injections. It goes through your body, driving out to the surface the diseases in the body and curing many more. But medicines you just swallow them and they go to your stomach. Injection is better" (182). Sleeping sickness is one of the illnesses that modern treatment has proven itself more effective than the traditional. When Sunsaye is bitten by a fly, struggling to kill it, Baba tells him, "It is the tsetse fly. It causes the sleeping sickness" (35). Some days after he gets contaminated, he is seen "wrapped in the thickest cloths. He was shivering and blubbering in his delirium" (*BG*, 44). Instead of being brought to the hospital, he is given traditional treatment: "Hodio handed him a concoction which he sipped greedily" (45). When the villagers ran away from the Whiteman, who offers health services in the village, Sunsaye says, "But you have not the sleeping sickness. . . . I heard that he gives the needle only to people with the sleeping sickness" (19). As a result, injection is effective in healing sleeping sickness and eradicating its germs. To protect the people from the sickness in Old Chanka, the white officials displace them to another village, newly named New Chanka, where "there is a place where a man with the sleeping sickness may go for treatment" (44). Here, no one suffers from the sleeping sickness again because as it is said, "the place is very clean. . . . It is like a hospital". This implies that medical officials take active parts to safeguard environmental sanitation and reduce health disorders associated with poor environment.

In *SOT*, when the catechist catches fever, he

> drank the warm fever grass his wife had placed in front of him. . . . The following morning, the Catechist got up with a lot of difficulty. He had a terrible headache. His wife prepared more fever grass tea for him to drink with honey and he lay back on the bed unable to get up.
>
> (*SOT*, 54)

Fever grass, also referred to as lemongrass, offers an array of medicinal benefits. In this father's case, its usage aims at curing his fever. Honey is also known for its curative values; it protects the body against damage caused by bacteria and can be mixed with certain medicinal products like herbs to have more favourable results. In the Catechist's case, the cold intensifies. When Ndong is informed he has only taken fever grass, "he sent some malaria and headache drugs from his first aid box to the Catechist. The Catechist took the drugs and went back to bed and slept on till afternoon when he got up feeling much better" (*SOT*, 55). The first aid box is a trace of the colonial medical establishment in postcolonial African society. It intends to offer first treatment to patients before taking them to the hospital if they do not get better. This is similar to the general care services provided to patients by non-specialized healthcare providers in traditional societies. This joint healing system clearly indicates that beyond the obliteration of colonial presence in postcolonial medical realities in Africa, medical postcolonialism combines the benevolent aspects of orthodox and traditional medicines in forging sustainable holistic medical practices in postcolonial Africa.

Conclusion

This chapter shows that despite the introduction of the medical sciences and its associated orthodox medicine in Sub-Saharan Africa, traditional healers continue to make a significant contribution towards holistic healing in postcolonial Africa. The African traditional medicine is the indigenous system of healthcare and it is holistic, in the sense that it heals both physical and spiritual illnesses. With the archaeological approach of literary texts, traces where they dispense healing through divination, herbalism, and spirituality were analysed. In traditional medicine, midwifery service providers give prenatal care to expecting mothers, attend to the birth of their infants, and provide post-partum care to the mother and her infant. Through medicine men's active role in safeguarding African identity through holistic healing, they are looked upon as guardians of traditional codes of morality and values. The characters have great faith in traditional medicine particularly because of the inexplicable aspects that it is the wisdom of their forefathers which also recognizes their socio-cultural and religious background. Therefore, besides the easy accessibility to traditional healers, traditional medicine provides an avenue through which cultural heritages are preserved and respected. African traditional medicine continues to be a relevant form of primary healthcare especially, in rural communities despite the existence of conventional orthodox medicine. In the context of health financing, traditional healers help to safeguard the lives of many Africans who cannot afford the cost of orthodox medicine. However, orthodox medicine in some ways is complementary to traditional medicine in postcolonial Africa. Modern hospitals may deal with the physical side of diseases, but there is the religious dimension of suffering which they do not handle, and for that purpose a great number of patients will resort to both hospitals and medicine men without a feeling of contradiction. In postcolonial Africa, both systems of medicine exist in the lives of the people, both have the primary objective to cure, manage or prevent diseases, and maintain good health. This portrays new attitudes enhanced by the contacts between bearers of many mentalities, in accordance with Edouard Glissant's call for a rhyzomatic identity.

References

Abdullahi, A.A. (2011). Trends and Challenges of Traditional Medicine in Africa. *African Journal of Traditional Complementary and Alternative Medicines*, 8: 115–123. Department of Sociology South Africa.

Ateh, F. (2018). *Seat of Thorns*. Cameroon: Nyaa Publishers.

Ekaney, J. (2007). *Verdict of the Gods*. Cameroon: Buma Kor Publishers Ltd.

Ekeopara, C. and Azubuike, U. (2017). The Contributions of African Traditional Medicine to Nigeria's Health Care Delivery System. *Journal of Humanities and Social Science*, 22(5): 32–43. www.iosrjournal.org. Accessed 24 December 2022.

Ekwensi, C. (1962). *Burning Grass*. London: Heinemann.

Faleye, O.A. and Akande, T.M. (2019). Beyond "White Medicine": Bubonic Plague and Health Interventions in Colonial Lagos. *Gesnerus: Swiss Journal of the History of Medicine and Sciences*, 76(1): 90–110.

Glissant, E. (1997). *Poetics of Relation* (trans. Betsy Wing). Michigan: The University of Michigan Press.

Liverpool, J. (2004). Western Medicine and Traditional Healers: Partners in the Fight Against HIV/AIDS. *Journal of the National Medical Association*, 96(6). Atlanta, Georgia.

Magesa, L. (1997). *African Religion: The Moral Traditions of Abundant Life*. Nairobi: Paulines Publications Africa.

Mumo, P.M. (2009). The Psychological Aspects of African Healing. *Hekima: Journal of Humanities and Social Sciences*, 4(1): 62–69.

Mumo, P.M. (2012). Holistic Healing: An Analytical Review of Medicine-Men in African Societies. *A Journal of the Philosophical Association of Kenya, New Series*, 4(1): 111–122. Nairobi: University of Nairobi.

Ngetcham. (2022). *Pour une Critique Archeologique des Arts et des Lettres*. Finlande: Atramenta.

Nwapa, F. (1966). *Efuru*. Ibadan: African Writer's Series.

Orgah, A.E. and Orgah, O.J. (2015). Herbal Medicine in Nigeria: A Practice at the Clinical Crossroad. *South American Journal of Clinical Research*, 2(2). Tianjin, China.

Swantz, L. (1990). *The Medicine Man among the Zaramo of Dar es Salaam*. Uppsala: Mai Palmberg.

10 Necropolitics and the Expression of "Madness" in Nigerian Poetry

Solomon Awuzie

Introduction

Necropolitics as a concept can better be deplored to describe the social-existential situation that is constantly reflected in postcolonial Nigerian poetry where the differential value placed on people results in psychological problems for others. In the view of Mbembe (2019), necropolitics pushes victims of differentiation into the *death-world*. The term*death-world* represents the consequences of the differential values to human life which, according to Mbembe (2019), include death and insanity. This chapter pays particular attention to how insanity, which is one of the consequences of necropolitics, has been prominently reflected in postcolonial Nigerian poetry. This chapter posits that it reflects in the outlook of the assertions of "madness" in poetry, hence literary critics' assumptions that some Nigerian poets are also "disturbed" (Oyebode, 2009: vii; Onyema, 2012: 41). Part of the reason for this is that postcolonial Nigerian poetry records the persona's traumatic and chaotic socio-political life and engages on how these have affected his emotional and mental well-being without relegating the madden government policies responsible for the disparities between people. Postcolonial Nigerian poetry is a very important platform from where the victim-persona's differential experience reflects in his poetic propositions as well as constitutes part of his neuroses. In his article on "Ecotrauma", Onyema (2012: 41) corroborates this view by insinuating that the victim-persona is not just a symbolic victim of his socio-political milieu but exhibits the behavioural codifications of a neurotic.

Being part of the postcolonial hegemonic discourse, this chapter shows that in addition to the commonly divulged dimensions of necropolitics, postcolonial Nigerian poetry explores the psychological realities of necropolitics among the Nigerian people. This chapter also reveals that there is a proliferation of the symptoms of madness in Nigerian poetry. While some poems reflect on the persona's neurosis, others engage with the schizophrenic as well as the paranoiac consequences of the persona's stay in a society where he is the victim of government differentiation. In the chapter, the contrast between the poems with the symptoms of schizophrenia and those with the symptoms

DOI: 10.4324/9781003429135-15

of paranoia is stressed. It is revealed that the symptoms of schizophrenia have dominance in the poetry of the older generations of Nigerian poets, while the symptoms of paranoia are evident in the poetry of the younger generation of Nigerian poets.

Through the analysis of the selected postcolonial Nigerian poetry, the inherent behavioural codifications in the poetry provide the reasons for the disparities between the symptoms that are diagnosed in the different poets. The chapter does not only link the persona's neurosis to the stress caused by the preference of others to him in his chaotic socio-political milieu but reflects on how his poetry has become a narcotic: the only measure that is necessary to return him back to the lane of sanity. In order to achieve this, this chapterhas been subdivided into five sections. While the introduction is meant to introduce the argument, the second and the third subsections engage with the important issues associated with necropolitics and postcolonial Nigerian poetry. In the fourth subsection, different postcolonial Nigerian poetry are analysed to depict the neurotic consequences of necropolitics on the victim-persona, and the fifth subsection concludes the argument. In it, inference is drawn from the entire discourse to reflect on the implications of the persistent diagnosis of the symptoms of insanity in postcolonial Nigerian poetry.

Necropolitics: Its Origin and Relationship With the Postcolonial Nigerian Poetry

Necropolitics is a term that is coined from the Greek root word "nekros", which means "corpse"; hence necropolitics simply translates to "the politics of death". Necropolitics was coined, introduced, and defined by its exponent, Achille Mbembe, in his 2003 article, as the ability to say who is important and who is not, "who is disposable and who is not". Mbembe understands necropolitics to include not just people experiencing death but people experiencing social or political death such as people suffering from insanity. People who are unable to set their own limitations because of social or political interference such as the insanity are considered not to be truly alive, because they do not have sovereignty over their own body. The ability for a state to subjugate populations so much so that they lost the liberty of autonomy over their lives or become insane is an example of necropolitics (see Umezurike 2018). Necropolitics creates zones of existence for the insane, those who no longer have sovereignty over their own body. As a theory, it refers to the use of social or political power to differentiate who is to die or who is to live, who is to be sane and who is to be insane. The term "necropolitics" gave birth to another term referred to as *death-world*, a term which Mbembe, in his book on necropolitics published in 2019, explained as a form of social existence where people are subjected to the experience that is similar to the condition of the living dead.

Necropolitics is an extension of Michel Foucault's concept of biopower and biopolitics, which were first discussed in Foucault's book titled *The Will to Knowledge: The History of Sexuality* Volume 1, published in 1976. In his book, Foucault describes biopower as the use of social and political power to control people's lives. He argues that biopower is a mechanism for protecting people but this protection manifests as subjugation of no-normative populations. While commenting on the fact that Foucault's concepts of biopower and biopolitics do not have the capacities to cover contemporary state-sponsored death, Mbembe notes that necropolitics, which is also called necropower, closes the lines between resistance and suicide, sacrifice and redemption, martyrdom and freedom. In response to the disparities between Foucault's biopolitics and Mbembe's necropolitics, Puar (2017) maintains that the discourse must be intertwined because the two are woven around each other. According to him, necropolitics introduces itself as the limits as a result of the loophole of biopolitics, while biopolitics "masks the multiplicity of its relationship to death and killing in order to enable the proliferation" of necropolitics (Puar, 2017: 66). Mbembe (2019) explains that the concept of necropolitics is particular about those he referred to as the "living dead". By the "living dead" Mbembe (2019) says that it is the condition in which people are made to remain in a suspended state of being between life and death. The concept of necropolitics is not only about the right to kill, it includes different forms of political violence which include the right to impose mortal danger, such as insanity, on others. Lauren Berlant (2007: 752) prefers to call this process of imposing mortal danger on others or the process of elimination, which are the core principles of necropolitics, "slow death". R. Guy Emerson (2019: 2) writes that necropolitics exists beyond the limits of administrative or state power being imposed on bodies, but also becomes internalized, coming to control behaviours over fear of death or fear of exposure to death worlds.

As a theory, necropolitics has always been deplored in the discussions of postcolonial Nigerian poetry without any particular mentioning of the term. It has always been linked to the reason for the manifestation of the symptoms of insanity in postcolonial Nigerian poetry and to underscore Nigerian poetry as the product of the poets' mental stress and anxiety. In his book entitled *Mindreadings: Literature and Psychiatry*, Professor of Psychiatry Femi Oyebode (2009) discloses that poetry does not only show the consequence of human reactional behaviours towards the fear of death but it can be deplored to reinforce the importance of poetry as psychotherapy. He illustrates that "like every other skill, our moral imagination, that is, our empathy, needs to be exercised and tested" and that poetry provides asafe way to do it (p. viii). The book also maintains that poetry can be an avenue to read the persona's mind as well as to showcase the persona's experience of necropolitics. However, it was the initial act of trying to read the persona's mind through the wordings of poetry that led to the erroneous assumption that the poet is also a madman. Despite the erroneousness of the argument, it dominated the earlier perception of the poet and has continuously fuelled contemplation on whether poetry should be counted as a true reflection of the human reactional behaviour towards the fear of death. This assumption has further given vent to the popular assertion that the radical influence of poetry is to be found across the entire spectrum of pathology. Part of the reason for this is that the poet takes his worriment to mind and later expresses them in his poetry. His lack of adaptation to the socio-political situation of his country is reflected in his poetry in the form of neurosis, schizophrenia and paranoia.

Among these three conditions, neurosis has been persistently described as the most common. Neurosis reflects on Nigerian poetry in the form of the poet's anxiety and distress. It is an automatic unconscious poetic effort to manage deep anxiety. The poetic behaviour is usually within the socially acceptable norms and may include anxiety, worry, negative as well as obsessive thoughts. A more sever poetic condition is schizophrenia. It reflects in Nigerian poetry in the form of a disorder in which the persona interprets reality in the poetry abnormally. It is a chronic disorder and it affects the way the persona expresses emotions, and perceives reality. The schizophrenic poetry may reflect what is called delusion as well as hallucinations. Poetry containing the experience of delusions may show the poet's belief that something is true when there is no strong evidence for it while the poetry containing the experience of hallucinations may report that the poet hears voices and see, feel, taste, or smell things that are not really there. For this reason, the poetic thought as well as the poetic line of a schizoid poetry may jump from one subject to another for no logical reason. It may therefore be hard to follow what the poetry is trying to say. Schizophrenia can first appear in the form of poetic depression. In contrast to depressivepoetry, schizophrenic poetry is characterized by reluctance, even an inability, to make human contacts – a disability which we have even seen in Nigerian poetry.

The Poet, His Poetry and the Debate on His Insanity

Despite the fact that the poet's experience of necropolitics has led him to produce poetry that reflect insanity is it right to assume the poet is a madman? In trying to answer this question Plato in "The Ion" (1986: 18) specifically identifies him as a madman. Sandblom (1989) corroborates Plato's postulation by recounting the experiences of the poets named Christopher Smart and Handel. According to him, these poets were confirmed to be insane and their mental conditions helped them in the production of great poetry. If this is true, does it mean that poets are spoken to be some demons like the schizophrenic and conditioned to put what he is told down in writing? If this is also true can we say that the Nigerian poet Ebereonwu (2004), who claimed he was inspired by some familiar demons, named "Medemede", into writing poetry, is a madman?

This familiar demon, which I have recognized by name as Medemede, has been doing overwork on me for a long time because some of the works here precede my first published work. Unlike other demons that intrude into the mind of a host against his will, Medemede is initially welcome by a writer. But caged, its presence in the form of a manuscript begins to appear like an intrusion. The writer wants it to go away and be published. But if a published contract would not come on time to provide leeway for an escape, Medemede begins to behave like a caged guest. And soon begins to distort the writer's view of himself and environment. Observing the distinction in the countenance of a published writer and a manuscript carrier, it is easy to understand who is at the greater mercy of Medemede, the demon of writing.

(12)

These perceptions of the poets as madmen have been debunked by scholars such as Charle Kaplan (1986), Sigmund Freud (1986), Lionel Trilling (1974) and Carl Jung (1971). In his book titled *Criticism: The Major Statements*, Kaplan (1986: 419) posits that the poet is not mad, but rather he is unsatisfied with the situation around him. Sigmund Freud (1986), in his famous essay titled "Creative Writers and Day-Dreaming", explained that the poet is not mad but that mental activity such as poetry is engaged towards inventing situations where his unsatisfied wishes are fulfilled. He notes that everyone has the creative impulse in him, but it is when the creative activity in the mind of an individual becomes too heavy that the individual loses touch with reality. Trilling (1974: 2805) shows a distinction between the illusions of the madman and the illusion of the poet by stressing that the illusion of the madman is physically disturbing, while the illusion of the poet is beneficent.

In his essay "On the Relation of Analytical Psychology to Poetry", Carl Jung (1971) agrees that the capacity to be troubled or to be unsatisfied with the situation around him distinguishes the poet from the rest of other individuals. Jung (1971: 322) explains this thus: "the normal man can follow the general trend without injury to himself but the poet takes to the back streets and alleys because he cannot endure the broad highway". Jung explains further that the contents of the "personal unconscious" and sometimes that of the "collective unconscious" are present in everyone but are resourceful to the poet. Poetry receives "tributaries from these spheres" only if they can mature into what he called an "autonomous complex". If not, what is received from the "personal unconscious", for instance, becomes a "muddy" poetry and "their predominance, far from making poetry a symbol, merely turns it into a symptom" (p. 319). And by "autonomous complex" he meant "a psychic formation that remains subliminal until its energy-charge is sufficient to carry it over the threshold into consciousness" (p. 317). What this implies is that what Ebereonwu referred to as "Medemede" is nothing but what Jung referred to as the "autonomous complex". What it means is that Ebereonwu writes through the help of the energy charge that is withdrawn from the conscious control of his personality. "Medemede", as Ebereonwu prefers to call his "autonomous complex", is not a spirit but the energy charge that feeds his creative complex. To other poets, the "autonomous complex" inspires the poetic creation but in Ebereonwu's case it has been different: the complex becomes tyrannical if there is no publishing contract for an already finished work. From Ebereonwu's description of the characteristics of Medemede, it is also responsible for the poet's ability to absorb what is happening around him.

Poetry and the Victim-Personas' Madden Expressions

Different postcolonial Nigerian poetry has different necropolitical rendition that reflects on the persona as neurotic, schizophrenic or paranoiac. Part of what tailors the poetry along this part is how the poet is able to manipulate his persona's musing to capture his painful life experience as well as engage his chaotic national experience. Through the help of his persona, the poet also engages with the different Nigerian people's maddened/unsatisfied utterances and behaviours. The poems of the older Nigerian poets were the first to set Nigerian poetry on the path of this revelation where poetry is reflected upon as the product of the poets' neuroses. Among the Nigerian poets whose poetry leads the way in this psychological reassessment is Christopher Okigbo. In Okigbo's *Labyrinths and the Path of Thunder* the persona's poetic utterances and his imaginary description of events have the outlook of schizophrenia. For instance, Okigbo's early poetry which was initially accused of obscurantism (see Chinweizu, Jemie, and Madubuike, 1980) has shown the persona's repeated inability to make human contact, as typical of the schizophrenic. As a poet, Okigbo was aware of the aberrant poetic behaviour that distinguishes poetry from other genres of literature; hence he decided to act it out when, as his brother Pius Okigbo (2008:ix) narrates, he "agreed to travel to Kampala, Uganda, for a conference of writers at the expense of the organizers only to mount the rostrum and refuse to read his poetry to non-poets." This goes to show that aberrant psychic traits which in ordinary people would seem morbid may add to the originality and infatuation of poetic creation; they may even constitute its basis or origin. Of course, Okigbo's aberrant psychic trait is evident in his early poetry which appears incomprehensible and inconceivably malicious. Okigbo's schizophrenic tendencies are first reflected upon in "The Passage", where the persona addresses a watery presence which he refers to as "mother Idoto". The poem indicates that the persona addresses a woman personage while standing before a river. In the poem, the persona wants his reader to believe that the river is either a woman which healone can see or is the abode of the woman. The persona claims that the imaginary woman has the human characteristics of hearing and perception; hence he yells in the later lines of the poem, thus: "out of the depths my cry:/give ear and hearken . . ." (1).

The poem can be interpreted as a window into the persona's mind and the activities of "mother Idoto" inthe later part of the poem are the reflections of the persona's illusions. Rather than having a violence consequence on the persona, the illusion of "mother Idoto" humbles him and helps him to undergo a psychic retreat to his African root. This retreat is later felt in Okigbo's "Path of Thunder", where the poems in the sequel engage the military activities that preceded the Nigerian Civil War. As typical of the schizophrenic, the relationship between Africans and the African gods that existed in the African past is relived in the persona's mind and is treated with some reverence. This African past as reflected in the persona's mind is exaggerated and complicatedly portrayed. He is able to describe "mother Idoto" underwater activities as well as make utterances that are not coherent. He says he is naked before Idoto's watery presence, and at the same time he claims to be leaning on an "oil-bean tree". The repeated appearance of rich symbols in the persona's mind means that his psyche is trying to communicate something other than the face-value fantasy. It is on this ground therefore that the symbolic word "naked" may not mean that the persona is without cloth and may suggest that the persona is undergoing purgation. However, there is a similar schizophrenic reflection in Wole Soyinka's poetry. In most of his poetry, Soyinka has persistently engaged a persona that can be diagnosed with paranoiac-schizophrenia.

Like Okigbo's persona, the persona that dominates Soyinka's poetry has in most cases been pictured in a state of hallucination where he narrates the activities of the Yoruba deity Ogun. In *Ogun Abibiman* for instance, Soyinka's persona does not only claim that he has the ability to behold Ogun, which is a spirit personage and its activities, but that Ogun is the deity of the entire black race and a brother to Dionysus. In the poem titled "Night" (see Senanu and Vincent, 1976: 119), Soyinka's persona contemplates night in the most schizophrenic manner. Not only did he describe nightfall as a woman but he also details its effect on him. He describes it as a woman who can be compared to a clam "on the sea's crescent" (p. 119). He claims that he saw the imaginary woman's "jealous eye quench the sea's/fluorescence" (p. 119). Even though it is illusionary for the persona to see a woman in the place of nightfall, it is also reflective of the persona's schizophrenic apprehension for him to state that the sea has a fluorescence which the woman's eye quenched. Through a series of images, the persona paints a picture of the "dawning" of the woman to whom he must submit. In the poem, there is an impression of self-identification and a hint on the woman's terror. However, whereas the persona in Okigbo's poetry as well as the one in Soyinka's poetry has the incline of hallucination, we see a different kind of schizophrenic reflection in Gabriel Okara's poetry, especially in his poem titled "The Call of the River Nun" (see Senanu and Vincent, 1976: 40). In the poem, Okara's persona complains of hearing voices. The voices, we are meant to believe, come in the form of a call. The persona tells the reader that the call which initially started off in a simple voice tone "gradually becomes complex and ends on a serious, meditative note" (Senanu and Vincent, 1976: 41). The persona notes that when it was just a call, he hears "it break the circle/of these crouching hills" (p. 40), but when it becomes a "lapping call", he hears "it come through;/invoking the ghost of a child/listening, where river birds hail/your silver-surfaced flow" (p. 40). In the poem, the message that comes with the call is incomprehensible and overtly impenetrable.

Interestingly enough we also see similar schizophrenic reflections among the second-generation Nigerian poets, but this only appears in a few poems that engage their personas' illusions about military despotism in the Nigerian political arena. As an important second-generation Nigerian poet, Tanure Ojaide's poetry is reflective of his persona's neurotic engagement. The poetry engages both Ojaide's perception of the chaotic national experience and his Niger-Delta experience. In "When soldiers are diplomats", the second poem in Ojaide's (1990) collection entitled *The Fate of Vultures and Other Poem*, the persona's neurotic utterances are in full displace. He refers to the soldiers as diplomats, and yet their diplomatic missions to the country are to deceive the populace, bring problems upon the nation and to kill its citizenry. In the poem the persona shows a high level of stress and anxiety. This may be as a result of his worries occasioned by the continuous stay of military despots in power. The tension in the poem is further stressed as the persona paints a picture of the soldiers in power as not just pretenders but very dangerous.

The poem also captures the persona's neurotic yeaning in the three major lines of the first stanza, thus: "you will never see the leopard's fangs in the dark/you will never trace the rainflushed blood trail to a den/you will never catch the slayer by his invisible hand" (p. 4). "The leopard's fangs in the dark", "the rainflushed blood trail to a den" and "the slayer by his invisible hand" are reflective of misplaced juxtapositions of a neurotic and differentiate Ojaide's persona from the schizophrenic persona that is encountered in Okigbo's poetry. Since neurotic utterances are dominated by irony, we see more of it in the poem. The ironic poetic lines "The bedbug doesn't care/for the taste of your blood" (p. 4) are evidence that the persona is stress torn. In the poem, the persona stresses the wickedness of the soldiers by symbolically representing them as "bedbug". The "bedbug" shows that the persona is unable to cope with the soldiers being at the herm of the country's political affairs. The poem is also dominated by the persona's fear about the activities of the soldiers. This fear is strongly evident in the lines which read thus: "The bedbug doesn't care/for the taste of your blood" (p. 4) and" . . . the bedbug, that smug cannibal,/doesn't care for the rank smell of blood" (p. 5). Apart from revealing the state of the persona's fear, the lines also show that the persona is unhappy about the situation. The poem captures the persona in a state where he is incapacitated: he fears the involvement of the military in the country's political affairs, yet he is unable to do anything about it. This is an indicator that the persona's mind is dominated by the illusion of the inadequate self. The inadequate self is a reflection of the persona's troubled miniature face lost in his giant human profile. Apart from Ojaide's poetry, this neurotic rendition is also evident in Ada Ugah's poetry.

In the poem titled "The Ballad of the Town-Crier" (Ugah, 1991: 4) Ugah's persona evokes his inadequate self-neurotic rendition. The persona feels it is not yet time for the country to prosper. Part of the reason for this is because the military was in power. At the part VIII of the poem, the persona refers to the military officers in power as "predators" (p. 6). In every line of the poem, the persona shows that he is mentally stressed and anxious for a better Nigerian state. As the poem progresses, the stress and anxiety take a different turn; it transforms into fear. In the poem one notices the invocation of the archetype of the "shadow". Just as Jung has rightly explained, the shadow is the side of our personality which we do not display in public. The persona presents the shadow of himself as a town-crier. This representation is occasioned by the fact that he is the poet whose major function is to inform the people. Unlike Ojaide and Ugah's different poetry that reflect on the neurotic rendition of their personas, the poetry of Isidore Diala and Hyginus Ekwuazi have shown the persona's paranoiac tendencies. In Diala's *The Lure of Ash* (1997) the persona's paranoiac tendency is evident in his treatment of the theme of the Nigerian Civil War. Part of the reason why this kind of psychological rendition is noted in the poem is because the collection tends to be sympathetic with the Biafran side. In the last subsection of the collection titled "The trail of ash", the persona "reflects on Amadioha as the symbol of the Biafran army. Amadioha in the Igbo pantheon is a god of justice and of a consuming fire: it protects the morally upright supplicant and avenges the wrong that is done to him" (see Awuzie, 2021: 3).

In the poem titled "The Priest and the Pilgrim" the persona is agitated. He describes Amadioha as the Biafran Army that is capable of killing many federal Nigerian soldiers if provoked. In the poem, the persona is portrayed as being critical towards the war, and this goes to show that he is infuriated by it. The persona imagines he could overturn the course of time where the Biafra militia group wins the federal forces. This is one of the reasons he chose to recreate the Biafra militia soldiers as Amadiaha whose "white light" is enough to cause countless death. The poem is filled with anger and frustration and the persona is constantly in a state of aggressiveness. We have also seen a similar paranoiac reflection in Hyginus Ekwuazi's poetry. Like Diala's poetry, Ekwuazi's poetry shows that suffering and pain could also be a muse. In *The Monkey's Eyes*, Ekwuazi's (2009) persona engages the happenings in Nigerian hospitals in the most paranoiac rendition.

In the preface to the collection, Ekwuazi himself tells us that the collection is about "a patient-persona who journeys through the hospital: through its rites and its rituals of healing; through the schedules and the protocols of its bureaucracy: and through the stress and strain of its restrictions" (p. 6) in the most torturous expedition. As the persona journeys through the wards of the hospital, the state of Nigerian hospital is anxiously and sadistically bemoaned. The persona's lamentation as well as his paranoiac dissatisfaction about the state of Nigerian hospital is first seen in the very first poem of the collection titled "Why doesn't a death sentence deafen the ears?" The persona paints the picture of Nigerian hospital where the death of patients is hastened. In the poem, the persona attacks both the doctors and the government.

He claims that most Nigerian doctors are careless about patients' life. This is evident in the lines where he states thus: "while he managed to remain untouched, totally/untouched . . . I was to him no more than a/mathematical problem that he must couch in the language/of a weather report" (p. 14). This indicates that Nigerian doctors are involved in guesswork during medical administration, and this has caused a lot of death.

Conclusion

From the analysis of the poetry, it has been shown that there are different psychological reflections in Nigerian poetry which are the evidence of necropolitical situation in Nigeria. From our analysis of different poems, we noticed special psychological features. While some poems reflect on the persona's schizophrenic inclines, others engage with the persona's neurotic as well as paranoiac renditions. The symptoms of schizophrenia are diagnosed in the poetry of the older generation of Nigerian poets because of their engagements with cultural battles with the white intellectuals. Using their poetry, African/Nigerian poets struggle to prove that African/Nigerian cultures matter by displaying heavy schizophrenic (schizoid) symptoms. The schizoid Nigerian poetry seeks the meaning of life which others find in human community. The poetry depicts the need for close personal contacts and the need to be liked and appreciated, For fear of being rejected, it shows that there is the need for recognition and this need is strongly stressed in the poetry. The schizoid persona of the first-generation Nigerian poetry feels that he has managed to restore the lines of communication to a lost world. Schizoid poetry have indicated the essential symptoms of the two psychopathologic temperaments which prevail in poet personas: the melancholy of the manic-depressive and the panic fear of the schizoid.

The personas of the second-generation poets such as Ojaide and Ugah portrayed the general neurotic inclination. Their poetry also shows that their personas are stress torn and overtaken by anger and frustration. The psychological reflection of the persona of younger generation poets such as Diala and Ekwuazi reveals the proliferation of the symptoms of paranoia. Diala and Ekwuazi's personas' paranoiac reflections go a long way to stress the high level of chaos in the Nigerian socio-space and harp on the need for Nigerian poetry to engage with the social and political violence that is responsible for the differentiation in the Nigerian socio-political space.

References

Awuzie, S. (2021). Grief, Resurrection and the Nigerian Civil War in Isidore Diala's the Lure of Ash. *Tydskrif vir Letterkunde*, 58(2). https://doi.org/10.17159/tlv58i2.6793.

Berlant, L. (2007). Slow Death. *Critical Inquiry*, 33(4): 752–762.

Chinweizu, J.O. and Madubuike, I. (1980). *Decolonization of African Literature.* Enugu: Fourth Dimension Publishing Co Ltd.

Diala, I. (1997). *The Lure of Ash.* Enugu: Nok Publishers International.

Ebereonwu. (2004). *The Unpublishable Poems.* Ibadan: KraftBooks Limited.

Ekwuazi, H. (2009). *The Monkey's Eyes.* Ibadan: Kraft Books Limited.

Foucault, M. (1978). *The Will to Knowledge: The History of Sexuality* (Vol. 1). London: Penguin.

Freud, S. (1986). Creative Writers and Day-Dreaming. In Kaplan, C. (Ed.), *Criticism: The Major Statements* (pp. 419–428). New York: St. Martin's Press.

Guy Emerson, R. (2019). *Necropolitics: Living Death in Mexico* (pp. 2–3). New York: Springer.

Jung, C. (1971). On the Relation of Analytical Psychology to Poetry. In Campbell, J. (Ed.), *The Portable Jung* (pp. 301–322). New York: The Viking Press.

Kaplan, C. (1986). *Criticism: The Major Statements.* New York: St. Martin's Press.

Mbembe, J.A. (2003). Necropolitics. *Public Culture*, 15(1): 11–40.

Mbembe, J.A. (2019). *Necropolitics.* Durham: Duke University Press.

Ojaide, T. (1990). *The Fate of Vultures and Other Poems.* Lagos: Malthouse Press Ltd.

Okigbo, C. (2008). *Labyrinths and Path of Thunder.* Lagos: Apex Books Limited.

Onyema, C. (2012). Ecotrauma, Dis-Locations, Dis-Eases and Global Parables in Chika Uniqwe's the Phoenix. *Ogele* (Special Edition), 2: 41–58.

Oyebode, F. (2009). *Mindreadings: Literature and Psychiatry.* London: RCPsych Publications.

Plato. (1986). The Ion. In Kaplan, C. (Ed.), *Criticism: The Major Statements* (pp. 17–20). New York: St. Martin's Press.

Puar, J.K. (2017). *Terrorist Assemblages: Homonationalism in Queer Times* (pp. 32–79). Durham: Duke University Press.

Sandblom, P. (1989). *Creativity and Disease: How Illness Affects Literature, Art and Music.* Philadelphia: GB Lippincott Company.

Senanu, K.E. and Vincent, T. (1976). *A Selection of African Poetry.* London: Longman Group Limited.

Trilling, L. (1974). From Freud and Literature. In Brooks, C., Lewis, R.W.B., and Warren, R.P. (Eds.), *American Literature: The Makers and the Making (Book D): 1914 to the Present* (pp. 2804–2812). New York: St. Martin's Press.

Ugah, A. (1991). *Colours of the Rainbow.* Lagos: Kraft Books Limited.

Umezurike, U.P. (2018). Land of Cemetery: Funereal Images in the Poetry of Musa Idris Okpanachi. *Tydskrif Vir Letterkunde*, 55(2): 134–145. https://dx.doi.org/10.17159/2309-9070/tvl.v.55i2.1325.

11 Trumpism and the Necropolitics of the Covid-19 Pandemic

Implications and Relevance to the African Socio-political Ambience

Durojaiye Owoeye

Introduction

At the outset of President Donald Trump's presidency, it became clear that the American socio-political scene was set for a turbulent and controversy-laden ride, for at least four years. The cataclysm that Trump's presidency forebodes is the emergence of another face of republicanism in the American political-ideological spectrum, a trumping of the established order in the Republican conservative disposition and structure as events would later reveal. Trumpism, the ideological manifestation of Donald Trump's extreme conservative sentiment, would in recent times go on to generate the most controversial of policy-forming bastions in the annals of the presidency of the United States of America. The complexity though does not hide the factuality that Trumpism is a radicalization of the conservative ideology far beyond the comfort of the Republican establishment. David Livingstone Smith has this to say about Trump's ideological contiguity with Fascism: "His rhetorical style, the approach that he used in his speeches, not just the first one but almost all the ones after it, really conformed to the analysis of Nazi rhetoric that is presented in that paper to an extraordinary degree" (KPFK RADIO, 2017). So divisive is Trumpism that some Republicans, Never Trump Movement (Schwartz, 2023, *Rolling Stone*), chose not to identify with the Trumpian ideology, in order to express their disdain for what they believed was the dishonour-ing of the Republican Party. Their discomfort notwithstanding, Trumpism, with its concomitant intense leaning towards anti-conventionalism, became the norm in the American presidency between 2017 and 2021 and still constitutes a menace to conventional thoughts about morality in American politics. In the midst of Trump's supremely rightist agenda emanates the coronavirus pandemic, in which case a virulent disease comes face-to-face with an equally virulent ideology, Trumpism. The stage is then set for a no-holds-barred confrontation between a universalism that underlines the need to keep the world safe from human degradation and a personalism that is boisterous in its presumptuous belief in the uniqueness of the individual, asserting that, after all, "the real is the personal, i.e., that the basic features of personality – consciousness, free self-determination, directedness toward

DOI: 10.4324/9781003429135-16

ends, self-identity through time, and value retentiveness – make it the pattern of all reality" (*Encyclopedia Britannica*). That the identity of the individual shall be a subject of uniqueness is not a subject of acute antagonism, but that identity-ideological construction should be over-prioritized to the detriment of public safety is the bane of Trumpism in its face-off with the social urgency to rid the American life of the tragedy called Covid-19.

This chapter, in the light of Trump's desire to circumvent medical conventionalism even in the face of glaring deathly reverberations, is an interpretative, nay, theoretical passion to have a very gripping understanding of Donald Trump's response to the outbreak of the pandemic. Pursuant to doing this, the theoretical and doctrinal platform of necropolitics and variants of structuralism, all of which manifest biopower sensibilities, are deemed appropriate for a penetrating discerning about Donald Trump's claims, counterclaims, rebuttals, and even mendacities as the pandemic spreads its fatal tentacles through every inch of American society. This chapter, is, therefore, a zealous craving to have an intellectual and literary perception of the ideological fault-lines that developed in and enveloped Donald Trump's responses to the coronavirus plague in the light of the overarching self-absorption that is characteristic of Trumpism as a socio-political ideology that tries to wean itself off the conventionality of the apparent indisputable facts surrounding the pandemic by throwing up arguments, counter-arguments, and, in some ridiculous cases, outright lies, all in a bid to prove its redoubtable uniqueness as a political fortress.

The second phase of these biopolitical cogitations about the responses of Donald Trump to the Covid-19 crisis, albeit much leaner in scope than the Trump affair, is their connective tissue with the Nigerian and South African ambience. The Nigerian socio-political system has some semblance with the ideological and philosophical turmoil that is the torment of Donald Trump in addressing the coronavirus scourge. Nigerian politicians, especially since 1999, have been a source of policy summersaults, behavioural crudities, and illegalities due to their self-centred arrogance, which strikes a personality confluence in Donald Trump's desire to upturn conventional reasoning about governance. Indubitably, the Trump syndrome, or Trumpism, as is evident in Trump's reckless oversight over the USA during his presidency as the disease ravaged, has some implications for social and political saneness or otherwise in the administration of Nigeria over the years.

The South African Covid-19 regime is particularly vital as a point of rumination on Mr. Trump's American cogitation about the pandemic, because the catastrophe that trailed its invasion was most devastating in South Africa, of all African countries. This South African importance, as a reference for critiquing Mr. Trump's response to the disease, is due to the high rate of infections and fatalities in the country, and this prominence became exceptionally thought-provoking as a result of the Omicron variant of the pandemic that emerged in Botswana but was given the necessary attention by the very sensitive and pro-active South African anti-Covid-19 authorities. Despite the gloomy picture that was drawn by the fatal umbrella over the nation, the South African anti-coronavirus crusade was a bright message about the developed nature of the countries that are still being cloaked in the "developing" construct, countries of the South. Albeit it has to be said that in some little sense, the existence of some negative parallel with an area of Trump's response to this global strain on social development existed, which, unlike Trump, was not an intentional underestimating of the deathly wave that was concomitant with the emergence of the malady.

Necropolitics in the Power Psychology of President Donald Trump's Zest to Halt the Coronavirus Wave

Power psychology fundamentally defines the relationship between President Trump and Americans in the former's attempt to stem the tide of the monster in Covid-19. At the same time, the president owes the populace a duty to make the environment as disease-free as he possibly can. Presidential powers are sourced from legally determined institutions, some of which are subject to the vagaries of politics, and politics in the grip of a sitting president like Donald Trump is the consequence of various emotional dispositions, which are not subject to the judgmental guide of reason or reasonableness. After all, political engagement is purposed on victory, the Machiavellian style, reason, and unreason being swept aside in its trajectory. Consciously or otherwise, presidential powers determine the fate of many citizens, the rich and the poor inclusive, as legitimacy is bestowed on the subject exercising the powers. Invariably, sovereignty resides in the president, who, albeit circumscribed by the constitution, lords it over the people in all manner of thought and action. This exercise of sovereign authority is seminal to the conceptualization of necropolitics. Trumpism as an ideology of conservatism, but with some gulf from the mainstream conservative ideology in American politics, has acquaintance in an element of Mbembe's neopolitics due to its (Trumpism's) newness in the American political firmament, "colonial occupation" (Mbembe, p. 25), occupation being an intervention in the life of a people. By creating an anti-establishment face of conservatism (which is new), Trumpism, which mothered Donald Trump's entrance into American politics, is reflective of Mbembe's "colonial occupation" concept –

> a matter of seizing, delimiting, and asserting control over a physical geographical area – of writing on the ground a set of social and spatial relations. The writing of new spatial relations (territorialization) was, ultimately tantamount to the production of boundaries and hierarchies, zones and enclaves; the subversion of existing property arrangements; the classification of people according to different categories; resource extraction; and, finally, the manufacturing of a large reservoir of cultural imaginaries. . . . Space was therefore the raw material of sovereignty and the violence it carried with it. Sovereignty meant

occupation, and sovereignty meant relegating the colonized into a third zone between subjecthood and objecthood.

(Mbembe, pp. 25 and 26)

Indeed, Trumpism, the ideology that energizes Donald Trump to partly preside over the waste of American lives, emerges as a colonial ideology that has come to occupy part of the spatial identity of the Republican conservative region to the extent that he has succeeded in militarising to the extreme the identity of Republicanism to the chagrin of many members of the party. The bloody and very violent invasion of the Capitol by pro-Trump supporters on 6 January 2021 is a striking evidence of the violent raw material of sovereignty. In fact, Trumpism as a "colonial" philosophy that was responsible for the calamitous regime of the pandemic in the USA was/is occupying two spatial regions: the immediate Republican Party and the macro-American society. The philosophy so much undermined the established Republican identity that still today, Donald Trump's grip on the soul of the party, though being flailed gradually (the result of the last midterm election a proof), is still substantially firm. That he could even gather so large size a vote in the 2020 presidential election is an attestation to his biopower control of a large space in the mega-American society.

Achille Mbembe conceives necropolitics as how

the ultimate expression of sovereignty resides, to a large degree, in the power and the capacity to dictate who may live and who must die. Hence, to kill or to allow to live constitute [*sic*] the limits of sovereignty, its fundamental attributes. To exercise sovereignty is to exercise control over mortality and to define life as the deployment and manifestation of power.

(Mbembe, 2003, p. 11)

One may not be able to controvert Mbembe's view about sovereignty because the exercise of sovereign power over life and death (especially concerning who to die and who to live), which lies with the president, though not overtly stated in any democracy, is an intrinsic prerogative of the American president. Against the backdrop of Donald Trump's responses to the coronavirus plague, which are immersed in the privatisation of politics and governance respecting Covid-19, sovereignty emerges indubitably "as a two-fold process of *self-institution and self-limitation* (fixing one's own limits for oneself)" (p. 13) (Italics not mine).

Ostensibly, Trump, in many of his decisions during the Covid-19 crisis, embodies a discomforting privatistic concern with power, power for the sake of the self, and not for the commonweal. He deploys, through the biopower style, the intricacies in public institutions for himself and, in the act, becomes a self-centred lord over executive limitations. He sets for himself, though covertly, advertently, and maybe more inadvertently, who to die and who to be saved during the pandemic. His proclivities towards the rich and the power-ful in the American socio-economic clime may have been responsible for this. The following cases countenance his inclination in this direction. Here is an instance of the president's bias as reported by the *New York Times,* and this is without prejudice to its repetition in the primary structuralist analysis of his responses later in this chapter:

> on February 24, hours before Trump declared on Twitter that the coro-navirus was of zero concern and that the stock market was looking hot, senior members of his economic team told wealthy and powerful members who sat on the board of the conservative Hoover Institution that things were much more precarious than the president had claimed.
> (Levin, 2020, *Vanity Fair*)

Using sovereignty to cloak his pro-rich prejudice and predilection, Trump has decided who to die and the converse, in which case, his rich friends, who have been apprised of the dangers of the scourge, would have taken appro-priate cautionary steps towards not contracting the virus, while the poor, who are being lied to by Trump, would feel complacent as a result of the president's assurances, and be ravaged by the health crisis. Trump's divergent pieces of advice now represent "the repository of death and terror as they equate sovereignty with a power to work by dynamics of 'selective elimina-tion'" (Das and Sahana, Book Review Excerpt, 2019) that necropolitics is all about.

The neopower functioning of sovereignty as resident in Trump also makes him pour accolades on some companies, who are busy profiting tremendously from presumably Trump's mercantilist passion in what Americans believed was his disastrous handling of the problem, which continued to kill Ameri-cans in droves: Writing for *Intelligencer,* Sarah Jones asserts thus:

> Trump's answer to a public health emergency [is] to enrich and empower the private sector. He used the occasion of his press conference to lavish praise on several corporations by name: the Swiss drugmaker Roche, which received an FDA patent for a COVID-19 test, and Thermo Fisher, an American company that will partner with the government to provide tests. From there the glad-handing only became more enthusi-astic. Trump thanked Google for "developing a website," upon which 1700 of its engineers are reportedly at work. (This is not quite true, as the Verge later reported. The website will be produced by a subsidi-ary of Google's parent company and will initially be available only in the Bay Area.) Dr Deborah Birx, who is overseeing the White House's coronavirus response, spoke glowingly of the government's "innova-tive response," which is "centered fully on unleashing the power of the private sector." That's great news for corporate executives, several

of whom were present for the press conference. Trump paraded them before the cameras, calling them "celebrities in their own right."

(Jones, 2020, Intelligencer)

This quoted passage accentuates the critical-mindedness of Mbembe about the capitalist erosion of the dignity of the have-nots and the underprivileged, the stratified sensibility of the mercantilist economic architecture, which incentivises Donald Trump's sovereign sentiment to glorify, albeit obliquely, the profiteering apparatus of the companies and his warning to the rich about the real horrors of the pandemic while lying to the deprived and destitute masses that all was well. Mbembe's neopolitics is reflective and penetrating about the rugged individualism, mercilessness, and brutal quest for pecuniary happiness and convenience of the capitalist orientation which Trump seems to glory and delight in, as he creates the plantation metaphor of the place of the disadvantaged and the impoverished in the American socio-political sphere:

There may, after all, be no reciprocity on the plantation outside of the possibilities of rebellion and suicide, flight and silent mourning, and there is certainly no grammatical unity of speech to mediate communicative reason. In many respects, the plantation inhabitants live non-synchronously. As an instrument of labor the slave has a price. As a property, he or she has a value. His or her labor is needed and used. The slave is therefore kept alive but in a *state of injury*, in a phantom-like world of horrors and intense cruelty and profanity. The violent tenor of the slave's life is manifested through the overseer's disposition to behave in a cruel and intemperate manner and in the spectacle of pain inflicted on the slave's body. Violence here become an element in manners, like whipping or taking of the slave's life itself: an act of caprice and pure destruction aimed at instilling terror. Slave life, in many ways, is a form of death-in-life. As Susan Buck-Morss has suggested, the slave condition produces a contradiction between freedom of property and freedom of person. An unequal relationship is established along with the inequality of the power over life. This power over the life of another takes the form of *commerce*: a person's humanity is dissolved to the point where it becomes possible to say that the slave's life is possessed by the master. Because the slave's life is like a "thing", possessed by another person, the slave existence appears like a perfect shadow.

(Mbembe, pp. 21 and 22) (Italicizing of the phrase
"state of injury" is not mine) (Italicizing
of the word "commerce" is mine)

Despite the commercialization trajectory that forces into being the inequality that is characteristic of the biopower situation, as apprehended in Trump's plaudits to the private sector, Mbembe does not deprecate the response of the "slave" with that of utter submission or self-denial but contends that, in some cases, the slave is capable of rebellion, as will be observable in one of his assertions very soon. Mbebe's resolution of the slave-master friction is apropos the "rebel" (Marcel, 2009, p. 261), "acceptance" (p. 32) and "nonacceptance" (p. 33) conceptual postulates of Gabriel Marcel's *homo viator* theory. Marcel, like Mbembe, brings up the "slave" consciousness in discussing the response of the oppressed. The rebel, in Marcel's perception, is this: "A slave who has received orders all life suddenly judges a command to be unacceptable" (p. 261), thereby expressing "nonacceptance" to the "slave" condition, the rebellion suggestion of Mbebe. The "acceptance" solution of the slave to the bondsman and bondswoman in Marcel's theorizing is the same as Mbembe's "suicide, flight and silent mourning". Unfortunately for President Donald Trump, the response of Americans to his graceless anti-Covid-19 performance smacks of the rebel and nonacceptance assumptions: the president lost his second-term bid, a result whose reverberations are still haunting the American socio-legal and political space.

Mbembe seems to be theoretically obliquely assertive about the American rejection of Donald Trump at the polls:

> In spite of the terror and the symbolic sealing off of the salve, he or she maintains alternative perspective over time, work, and self. This is the second paradoxical element of the plantation world as a manifestation of the state of exception. Treated as if he or she no longer existed except as a mere tool and instrument of production, the slave nevertheless is able to draw almost any object, instrument, language, or gesture into a performance and then stylize it. Breaking with uprootedness and pure world of things of which he or she is but a fragment, the slave is able to demonstrate the protean capabilities of the human bond through music and the very body that was supposedly possessed by another.
>
> (Mbembe, p. 22)

Without any gainsaying, the American people availed themselves of political instrumentality, political language, and political gestures to shut down the "terror" instrument of the erstwhile president.

The effect of Trumpism as an ideology on Donald Trump's responses to the scourge, when related to Mbembe's necropolitics, becomes more interesting a critique in the nexus between necropolitics and Michel Foucault's theory of biopower. To Foucault, biopower is produced from biopolitics, which

> refers to the Humanitarian values that deal with the political relations between the administration and or regulation of the life of species and a locality's populations, where politics and law can re-evaluate life based on constants and traits existing in the Natural [phenomenological] world.
>
> (Lemke, 2011, pp. 9 and 10)

Mbembe's expatiation of the biopower syndrome seems to spotlight Trump's prejudicial initiative in dealing with the pandemic. To Mbembe, biopower is "the domain of life over which power has taken control" (Mbembe, p. 12). Some questions he asked as a consequence of this definition enclose Trump's disastrous anti-Covid-19 administration in ideological *"deathworlds"*, Mbembe's word for the tragic upshot of neopolitics as the "use of social and political power to dictate how some people may live and how some must die" (Das and Sahana, Book Review Excerpt, 2019).

The following are the questions:

> But under what practical conditions is the right to kill, to allow to live, or to expose to death exercised? Who is the subject of this right? What does the implementation of such a right tell us about the person who is thus put to death and about the relation of enmity that sets that person against his or her murderer? Is [sic] the notion of biopower sufficient to account for the contemporary ways in which the political, under the guise of war, of resistance, or of the fight against terror, makes [sic] the murder of the enemy its primary and absolute objective? War, after all, is as such a means of achieving sovereignty as a way of exercising the right to kill. Imagining politics as a form of war, we must ask: What place is given to life, death, and the human body (in particular the wounded or slain body)? How are they inscribed in the order of power?
>
> (Mbembe, p. 12)

A punctilious scrutiny of these questions reveals the ideological and doctrinaire association of Trumpism and Trump's emotive connections with Mbebe's necropolitics. The first question borders on how Mbembe "draws on the concept of biopower and explores its relation to notions of sovereignty (*imperium*) and the state of exception" (Mbembe, p. 12). What is the state of exception? A state of exception is "similar to a state of emergency (martial law) but based on the sovereign's ability to transcend the rule of law in the name of the public good" (Kim, 2020, pp. 1001–1083). It is not in doubt that the pandemic was an emergency though one without martial law, and this is where Mbembe seems to shed light on the contradictions in democracies, democracies unravelling through the monstrosities of the negative use of power. Mbembe says much about the necropolitical nature of modern democracies:

> contemporary forms of democracies have ended up becoming necropolitical, though with their workings democracies have always reflected their constitutive biopolitical orientation. For him, necropolitics stands as a politics of "selective elimination" or negation of diverse blocs of masses that the state machinery considers resistant or redundant to its workings and policies, while biopolitics aims to control and govern the masses or better the dynamic expanse of life. If biopolitics yields what

is called "a control society" that engineers and subjects the masses to strategies of surveillance and control in order to govern them, necropolitics yields "a society of enmity". This happens to be a society that aims at altogether dispensing with the inherent revolutionary potential of masses by systematically and routinely decimating them – killing the poor to eradicate the rebellious discontentment of poverty and killing the powerless to form a tiny section of powerful elites, as one may say. Such a society feverishly creates new grounds or conditions propitious for strategical praxis of necropolitics. Further, as necropolitics works by turning death into a profitable industry, a society that becomes necropolitical ends up engineering death-making institutions only to treat masses as grist for the smooth working of these institutions.

(Das and Sahana, Book Review Excerpt, 2019)

As a democracy, America does not attract martial law during an emergency like the Covid-19 pandemic, "a state of exception". However, Trump, as a person wielding the power of sovereignty, "the right to kill", consciously or unconsciously, creates a martial law circumstance due to his negligence of the deadly viral situation, as he exposes, indirectly or directly, some people to living and others to dying.

The second question relates to who the subject of "the right to kill, to allow to live, or to expose to death" is. The subject in Trump's exercise of sovereign power is a personality that enunciates very clearly how the sovereign in modern states exploits the constitutionality of the sovereign to draw, consciously or otherwise, the fatal eliminatory agenda (who to live and die), underscoring Foucault's submission "that the right to kill *(droit de glaive)* and the mechanisms of biopower are inscribed in the way all modern states function" (Mbembe, p. 17). The sovereign in some modern states like America is restricted in the use of power but the person wielding the power is not absolutely restrained, as the constitution still gives the person a leeway through which some unconstitutionality (wishful decision about who to live) can be availed of. In a power-sensitive and mendacious character like Donald Trump, Mbembe's biopolitical "multiple concepts of sovereignty" (p. 13) can be discerned to give the democratic tyrant the all-clear to act unconstitutionally. Mbembe appraises the population of the democratic system and concludes, "These men and women are posited as full subjects capable of self-understanding, self-consciousness, and self-representation" (p. 13), but bound by "the ultimate expression of sovereignty [which] is the production of general norms by a body (the demos) made up of free and equal men and women" (p. 13). In other words, there are sets of laws that guide the citizenry, yet the leaning towards the self by the citizens may blunt and cripple some aspects of the constitution pursuant to satisfying narcissistic desires. The multiplicity of political sovereignty, which is realized in "a project of autonomy and the achieving of agreement among a collectivity through communication and recognition" (p. 13), is abused by Trump to invigorate his political sentiment over and above his constitutional duty of protecting all Americans.

The multiplicity of sovereignty having been identified as a neopolitical source of President Donald Trump's emotional devaluation of the democratic space during the pandemic, his obsession with the self is believed to have reached its adverse apogee when critiqued in the light of Mbembe's thesis on "Biopower and the Relation of Enmity" (p. 16). The ideology of hate unfortunately is the epicentre of Trumpism as a political ideology, a political philosophy that wants, to a high extent, the derogation of blacks particularly, and the minorities in general, in the American society, his doctrinaire obsession being of the white supremacist ontology. This interpersonal denigration is a subject of rumination in neopolitics as palpably communicated by Mbembe:

In Foucault's formulation of it, biopower appears to function through dividing people into those who must live and those who must die. Operating on the basis of a split between the living and the dead, such a power defines itself in relation to a biological field – which it takes control of and vests itself in. This control presupposes the distribution of human species into groups, the subdivision of the population into subgroups, and the establishment of a biological caesura between the ones and the others. This is what Foucault labels with the (at first sight familiar) term *racism*.

That race (or for that matter *racism*) figures so prominently in the calculus of biopower is entirely justifiable. After all, more so than class-thinking (the ideology that defines history as an economic struggle of classes), race has been the ever present shadow in Western political thought and practice, especially when it comes to imagining the inhumanity of, or rule over, foreign peoples. Referring to both this ever-presence and the phantomlike world of race in general, Arendt locates their roots in the shattering experience of otherness and suggests that the politics of race is ultimately linked to the politics of death. Indeed, in Foucault's terms, racism is above all a technology aimed at permitting the exercise of biopower, "that old sovereign right of death". In the economy of biopower, the function of racism is to regulate the distribution of death and to make possible the murderous functions of the state. It is, he says, "the condition for the acceptability of putting to death."

(pp. 16 and 17)

Reports from the States prove beyond reasonable doubt the factuality of Mbembe's identification of racism in the logic of biopower, as it is revealed "that minorities have been disproportionally affected by the pandemic. These minorities in the United States are not having their right to health fulfilled" (Reyes, 2020: 299), That the minorities "are not having their right to health fulfilled" supports the biopower view of the deliberate decision of the sovereign to tactically fatally eliminate some people. This calculated and cold-blooded intention to deny the minorities of social amenities, thereby leading to the highest rate of fatalities among them during the Covid-19 exigency in the USA under the sovereign watch of Donald Trump is hereby evidentially attested to:

> According to the World Health Organization's report *Closing the Gap in a Generation: Health Equity through Action on the Social Determinants of Health*, "poor and unequal living conditions are the consequences of deeper structural conditions that together fashion the way societies are organized – poor social policies and programs, unfair economic arrangements, and bad politics." This toxic combination of factors as they play out during this time of crisis, and as early news on the effect of the COVID-19 pandemic pointed out, is disproportionately affecting African American communities in the United States. I recognize that the pandemic has had and is having devastating effects on other minorities as well.
>
> (Reyes, p. 299)

In terms of specifics, African Americans, of the races, seem to be on the gloomiest platform of the pandemic's ravages, according to this established statistics:

> the data that are available highlight African Americans' overall lack of access to testing. For example, in Kansas, as of June 27, according to the COVID Racial Data Tracker, out of 94,780 tests, only 4,854 were from black Americans and 50,070 were from whites. However, blacks make up almost a third of the state's COVID-19 deaths (59 of 208). And while in Illinois the total numbers of confirmed cases among blacks and whites were almost even, the test numbers show a different picture: 220,968 whites were tested, compared to only 78,650 blacks.
>
> Similarly, American Public Media reported on the COVID-19 mortality rate by race/ethnicity through July 21, 2020, including Washington, DC, and 45 states. These data, while showing an alarming death rate for all races, demonstrate how minorities are hit harder and how, among minority groups, the African American population in many states bears the brunt of the pandemic's health impact. Approximately 97.9 out of every 100,000 African Americans have died from COVID-19, a mortality rate that is a third higher than that for Latinos (64.7 per 100,000), and more than double than that for whites (46.6 per 100,000) and Asians (40.4 per 100,000). The overrepresentation

of African Americans among confirmed COVID-19 cases and number of deaths underscores the fact that the coronavirus pandemic, far from being an equalizer, is amplifying or even worsening existing social inequalities tied to race, class, and access to the health care system.

(pp. 300 and 301)

With Donald Trump's many racist and prejudice-laden statements about American minorities, especially African Americans, there will be little controversy about the connexion between his White supremacist Trumpist ideology, one that may have aided his sovereign enabling of the death of more blacks than other races in his presidential fight against Covid-19, and the biopower political machinery of Achille Mbembe's necropolitics. Arguably and plausibly, President Donald Trump's Covid-19 struggles are a complete conflation of war and politics (Mbebe, p. 18), a vindication, indication, and demonstration of "terror formation" as a concatenation of biopower, the state of exception, and the state of siege" (p. 22).

Structuralism as a Complex Meaning-Dispersal Theory

It has to be prefigured that the structuralist instrument that will suffice in this analysis may be multipronged due to the multifaceted definitional structure of the theory as propounded by structuralist theorists of different hues. The structuralist explication of Donald Trump's engagement with the Covid-19 emergency will, therefore, be conducted through an all-inclusive face of the structuralist paradigm but taking into account the exigencies of clear-cut systemic distinctions so as to stave off an analytical process that is burdened by theoretical mix-ups. At all events, the complex Trump syndrome, the fount of the man's responses to issues, cannot but be critiqued from a multidimensional conceptual framework.

Structuralism in literature is one of the formalist attempts to undermine the homespun engagement with the literary enterprise, but like all other formalist theories, it ends up being a critical instrument for analysing the world outside the precincts of form-inclined literature. In its untainted and pristine or foundational form, the structuralist theory is a creation of Ferdinand de Saussure, "who was not interested in what people actually said (parole) but was concerned with the objective structure of signs which made them possible in the first place, and this he called langue" (Eagleton, 2008: 84). Structuralism, because of its concern with language, "attempts to apply the linguistic theory to objects and activities other than language itself" (p. 84) to the extent that one "can view a myth, wrestling match, system of tribal kingship, restaurant menu or oil painting as a system of signs" (p. 84). Essentially, Saussure's structuralism "viewed language as a system of signs, which should be studied 'synchronically' as a complete system at a given point in time, and not diachronically in its historical development" (p. 84).

At this juncture, the pseudo-structuralist principles of Northrop Frye will be examined, for in the analysis that will be done, some aspects of his structuralist thought will be of immense importance though within the structuralist Grundnorm of Sausure. Frye is convinced that in literature, there are "four narrative categories" of "the comic, romantic, tragic and ironic" (p. 80). Though these four categories are, in Frye's view, a platform for literary criticism, they can nonetheless be a medium to understand a non-literary phenomenon – after all, the non-literary narrative is structurally built like its literary counterpart, and if punctiliously analysed, the former can be appreciated to evince the structuration of the fictional narrative, as will be deciphered later in this analysis. This appreciative nexus between the literary and non-literary is made more realisable in Frye's theory of modes where the hero is described in the context of some genre manifestations; after all, is Trumpism, the political ideology that energises Donald Trump's responses to the medical predicament, not a "hero" personalisation of a character with a grand impression of himself? Frye contends that "Fictions . . . may be classified, not morally, but by the hero's power of action, which may be greater than ours, less, or roughly the same" (Frye, 1957: 33). By design, Trumpism, the provenance of Trump's turbulence-ridden anti-Covid-19 tutelage, is ideologically amoral in its cosmological denunciation of conventional or established moral expectations. Frye's fictive suggestions about the hero's might in genres are presented:

> If superior in *kind* both to other men and to the environment of other men, the hero is a divine being, and the story about him will be a *myth* in the common sense of a story about a god. . . . If superior in *degree* to other men and to his environment, the hero is the typical hero of *romance*, whose actions are marvellous but who is himself identified as a human being. The hero of romance moves in a world in which the ordinary laws of nature are slightly suspended. . . . If superior in degree to other men but not to his natural environment, the hero is a leader. He has authority, passions and powers of expression farer than ours, but what he does is subject both to social criticism and to the order of nature. This is the hero of the *high mimetic* mode, of most epic and tragedy. . . . If superior neither to other men nor to his environment, the hero is one of us: we respond to a sense of his common humanity. . . . This gives us the hero of the *low mimetic* mode, of most comedy and realistic fiction. . . . If inferior in power or intelligence to ourselves, so that we have the sense of looking down on a scene of bondage, frustration or absurdity, the hero belongs to the *ironic* mode.
>
> (pp. 33 and 34)

In the structuralist exploring of Trump's responses to the Covid-19 catastrophe, these senses of hero construction will be pivotal. These Trump's responses can also be conceived in terms of Frye's suggestion that in fiction (a reminder that fictive principles can be discoverable in real-life narratives) exists "a "comic" tendency to integrate the hero with his society, and a "tragic" tendency to isolate him" (54). That structuralism is concerned with structures, particularly with examining the general laws by which they work (Eagleton, p. 82), makes the structuralist application to appreciating Donald Trump's commitment to dealing with the Covid-19 exigency very appealing as social, medical, moral, and political mores are the references during the debacle. In this analysis, which is about confrontations with established concepts of thought, Frye's structuralist mentation continues to be of immense influence, as he "contrasts conservative 'myths of concern' with liberal 'myths of freedom', and desires an equable balance between the two (p. 81). To Frye, "the authoritarian tendencies of conservatism must be corrected by myths of freedom, while a conservative sense of order must temper liberalism's tendencies towards social irresponsibility" (Eagleton, p. 81). Without doubt, the conflict between "conservative 'myths of concern' and liberal 'myths of freedom'" expresses itself very vividly in Donald Trump's philosophy, "Trumpism", revealing a paradox in the workings of the ideology. This is simply due to the fact that Trumpism is first and foremost a conservative ideology with its own myths of concerns as distinct from the 'myths of concern' of the mainstream American conservative party. Secondly, and more functionally, Trump is deeply concerned with some myths of freedom as would extricate him from the conservative centre, and so the gap between him and the centre of Republican conservatism becomes widened, which takes its toll on his response to the Covid-19 implosion.

Being a quasi-structuralism, as is interpretable from the explication of modes and myths above, Frye's system of thought "deftly combines extreme aestheticism with a classifying 'scientificity'" (p. 81), which is revelatory in his systemic literary distinctions. An imitation of structuralism, Frye's work is suggested to be structuralist in the sense of its concern with structures but in a more or less loose framework due to the fact that "structuralism proper contains a distinctive doctrine which is not to be found in Frye: the belief that the individual units of any system have meaning only by virtue of their relations to one another" (p. 82). The relational concern with systems that underlies the traditional conception of structuralism will, therefore, be interpretatively functional in this discourse on Donald Trump and the medical explosion called coronavirus on the one hand, and its impact on the Nigerian socio-political environment on the other hand. In which case, "you become a card-carrying structuralist only when you claim that the meaning of each image is only a matter of its relation to the other" (p. 82). The relational reasoning in this structuralist exercise is cogently attested to in Soyinka's argument in his comparison of the Nigerian culture of lying with Trump's pathological inclining towards mendacity. Wole Soyinka argues in the foreword to *Trumpism in Academe*:

> While our own "dear native land" must claim credit for inspiring the sub-series *The Republic of Liars*. . . no suggestion was ever made – thank goodness! – that limited the catchment zone to our own national borders. Such an attempt would have been doomed from the start. There are challengers and – champions – elsewhere, seeking to wrest the laurels of lies from our own inspirational nation. Anyone in any doubt of this has only to refer to the daily record set within the United States in the past four years, all thanks to the industry of one man – her ex-president Donald Trump.
>
> (Soyinka, 2021:v)

Hence, as the analysis progresses, the pristine relational constitution of structuralism will no doubt be a domineering analytical force since the data collected shall be a subject of cross-referencing in the signifying process. Of course, it will be self-denial if this chapter will constrictively be about structuralism without the intrusive mechanism of post-structuralism coming into play to disentangle some structural opinions in this chapter on conceptual conflict, because structuralism itself, as theorized by Saussure, is self-deconstructive in its relational conclusions, though it is oblivious of the conceptual denial until Jacques Derrida postulated his counter-structuralist view of indeterminacy. In that event, the diachronic sensibilities of Derrida will indubitably unconsciously rein in the synchronic susceptibilities of Saussure at some junctures in this disquisition.

Understanding Saussure's structuralism brings into this analytical context the anti-conventionalism of Donald Trump, Saussure's structuralist thinking being a disavowal of the conventionality of meaning. Saussure's structuralism is based on the argument that the meanings of words are baseless creations of conventional thought. Saussure argues: "Each sign was to be seen as being made of a 'signifier' (a sound-image or its graphic equivalent), and a signified (the concept or meaning)" (Eagleton, p. 84). To Saussure, "The relation between signifier and signified is an arbitrary one: there is no reason why these three marks should mean 'cat', other than cultural and historical convention" (p. 84). Expounded, the argument is that

> The relation between the whole sign and what it refers to (what Saussure calls the "referent", the real furry four-legged creature) is therefore also arbitrary. Each sign in the system has meaning only by virtue of its difference from the others. "Cat" has meaning not "in itself", but because it is not "cap", or "cad" or "bat".
>
> (p. 84)

The siege on conventionalism and arbitrariness in ascribing meaning to objects by Ferdinand de Saussure parallels Donald Trump's counter-ideology against conventional Republicanism as a political ideology and as an "arbitrary" thought-system, which ineluctably impacts his responses to the novel coronavirus problem in the United States of America.

The reliance on difference and relational concerns makes Sausurre's structuralist approach a critical necessity in any scholarly event, depending on the analytical mindset of the critic. Saussure, it has to be said, "was not interested in what people actually said (parole) but was concerned with the objective structure of signs which made their speech possible in the first place, and this he called langue" (p. 84). This statement may be true to a large extent but it is not likely to be absolutely true in the light of the relatedness of signs which may be subjected to symbolic interpretations with the "referent" (the actual action) being the ultimate point of reference in any structuralist analysis. In this chapter, the relational trajectory of structuralist criticism is vital in that "[t]he relations between the various items of the story may be ones of parallelism, opposition, inversion, equivalence and so on" (p. 83). In this chapter, the four elements are indeed played out by Trump, the context being conflictual, with political repercussions.

Roman Jacobson of the Moscow Linguistic Circle is another notable theorist whose intellectualism helps to create a bond between Formalism and structuralism. His idea of the "poetic" is inherent in the postulation that language is "placed in a kind of self-conscious relationship to itself [thereby making it apparent that] The 'poetic' functioning of language 'promotes the palpability of signs" (p. 85). In other words, the linguistic techniques observed in a communication encounter create meaning. Without doubt, the language one uses is used to identify the probable signifying characters or human qualities that a person has. Roman Jacobson's six communication elements will also be instructive in this structuralist analysis as it progresses. The elements are: "an addresser, an addressee, a message passed between them, a shared code which makes that message intelligible, a 'contact' or physical medium of communication, and a 'context' to which the message refers" (p. 85). For the purpose of analytical clarity, Jacobson is discerning to note that in the communication arena, not all the elements may be functionally alive as "[a]ny one of these elements may dominate in a particular communicative act" (p. 85). This structuralist criticism is likely to be revealing in the light of this bias in Jacobson's communication concept. The world of equivalences as enunciated by Jacobson through metaphor and metonymy is another structuralist route to understanding the responses of Donald Trump to the coronavirus calamity. The issue of substituting words for others due to similarity as it exists in metaphors and the subject of word-association in metonymy will also be of importance in this attempt to understand more the politics that may undermine getting it right in a pandemic situation. Metaphor and metonymy are necessary in structuralism because of palpable signs in things that create contiguities in developing characters, and phenomena of like natures.

C. S. Peirce's semiotics is another structuralist instrument that will largely be of importance in this attempt to have cognition of the interesting dialogue between the politicization of medical realities and sustaining an extreme ideological conviction. The work of the Prague School of Linguistics makes structuralism to twin itself with semiology or semiotics, the latter being "the systematic study of signs [which is] what literary structuralists are really doing" (p. 87). Peirce's distinction between three kinds of signs will make it possible to analyse political and moral sentiments on the political-moral platform of this discourse. The signs are:

> the iconic, where the sign somehow resembled what it stood for (a photograph of a person, for example); the "indexical", in which the sign is somehow associated with what it is a sign of (smoke with fire, spots with measles); and the "symbolic", whereas with Saussure the sign is only arbitrarily or conventionally linked with its referent.
>
> (p. 87)

Other classifications will, of course, serve to augment those three signs in this exegesis. They are:

> "denotation" (what the sign stands for) and "connotation" other signs associated with it); between codes (the rule governed structures which produce meanings) and the messages transmitted by them; between the "paradigmatic" (a whole class of signs which may stand for one another) and the "syntagmatic" (where signs are coupled together with each other in a "chain"); It speaks of "metalanguages" where one sign-system denotes another sign-system (the relation between literary criticism and literature, for instance), "polysemic" signs which have more than one meaning.
>
> (pp. 87 and 88)

If "'structuralism' itself indicates a *method of enquiry*, which can be applied to a whole range of objects from football matches to economic means of production; [and] semiotics denotes a rather *field of study*, that of systems which would in an ordinary sense be regarded as signs: poems, bird calls, traffic lights, medical systems and so on [. . .]" (p. 87), the structuralist explication of President Donald Trump's responses to the medical catastrophe is likely to be worth the while. This is more so since structuralism and semiotics are entangled in the systematic study of signs as represented by human and non-human phenomena in their structural compositions.

The work of Yury Lotman, a Soviet semiotician, cannot be excluded in any structuralist construction as he "sees the poetic text as a stratified system in which meaning only exists contextually, governed by sets of similarities and oppositions" (p. 88). There is no gainsaying the fact that the Republican Party and the American presidency of Donald Trump's turbulence-laden response to the pandemic are inundated with ideas of variegated and hierarchy-sensitive predispositions and interests, and so the sympathies and antagonisms therein are of primary focus in a structuralist critical endeavour. Due to the stratified layers of interests in Lotman's semiotic reasoning, it turns out to be

> a system of systems, a relation of relations. It is the most complex form of discourse imaginable, condensing together several systems each of which contains its own tensions, parallelisms, repetitions and oppositions, and each of which is continually modifying all of the others.
>
> (p. 89)

Examining the Donald Trump American presidency reveals a complex web of actions and reactions, some of which influence the president's treatment of the pandemic.

For Lotman, analysing the text is also subject to external interpretations because

> The meaning of the text is not just an internal matter: it also inheres in the text's relation to wider systems of meaning, to other texts, codes, and norms in literature and society as a whole. Its meaning is also relative to the reader's "horizons of expectations".
>
> (p. 89)

In the same vein, the elements that function as the responses of President Donald Trump to the Covid-19 outbreak can be linked with issues external to them, for the president's response is in part a manifestation of his antiestablishment sentiments. In addition, the reader-response syndrome of I. A. Richards' *Practical Criticism*, from the reader's "horizons of expectations" perception, will be useful in the sense that the critic's interpretive thoughts have the carte blanche to revel in hermeneutic tolerance.

In that statement about meaning not being a monopolistic property of the internal workings of the text, Yuri Lotman is simply amplifying the intertextual nature of, in the primary sense, literature, and in the secondary sense, life, generally speaking. This intertextual quality of literature, or life, explains: "The literary work . . . is a continual generating and violating of expectations, a complex interplay of the regular and the random, norms and deviations, routinized patterns and dramatic defamiliarizations" (p. 89). These elements that generate and violate expectations are graspable in this structuralist interpretative venture. Fundamentally then, Lotman "does not consider that poetry or literature can be defined by their inherent linguistic principles", thereby undermining structuralism's primary formalist nature.

The narratological treatise of Gérard Gennete is believably a structuralist mode of apprehending the text or an issue, be it political, social or economic. Gennete conceptualizes "the distinction between *récit* by which he means the actual order of events in the text; *histoire*, which is the sequence in which those events 'actually' occurred, as we can infer from the text; and *narration*, which concerns the act of narrating itself" (p. 91). At some point in this analysis, this distinction will be needed for analytical clarification. Besides that distinction, Gennete's "five central categories of narrative analysis" will be a supplement to that *récit-histoire* difference. These categories are temporal in shape and they will be a guide concerning Trump's adventure into conflict and controversy respecting his attentions and dedications to the American public as it grapples with the Covid-19 virus. They are

"order" [which] refers to the time-order of the narrative, how it may operate by prolepsis (anticipation), analepsis (flashback) or anachrony, which refers to discordances between "story" and "plot". "Duration" signifies how the narrative may elide episodes, expand them, summarize, pause a little and so. "Frequency" involves whether an event happened once in the "story" and is narrated once, happened once but is narrated several times, happened several times and is narrated several times, or happened several times but is narrated once.

(pp. 91 and 92)

All these variegated tenets of structuralism will be invaluable in bringing into view how President Donald Trump's responses to the Corona pandemic shaped his presidency in part due to his ideological commitment to creating an extreme conservatism out of the conservative order of the Republican Party in the USA.

The Mediation of Structuralist Poetics Over President Donald Trump's Responses to the Coronavirus Calamity

The mediatory influence of structuralism in a scholarly attempt to put in perspective the responses of President Donald Trump is ". . .] a constant reminder of the etymological link between 'crisis' and 'criticism' " (Norris, 1991:x and xi). The crisis nature of the president's epileptic and febrile attitude to several aspects of the prophylactic and therapeutic requirements of the pandemic makes this chapter more compelling. The issue is so critical not just because it impacts very turbulently on the health of Americans but also due to the aura of confrontations, confusion, and complexities that it engenders over governance. Hence, the work of the critic becomes very crucial in interpreting one way or another how the entanglements created by the Trump-Covid-19 conflict place a huge burden on socio-ideological and political understanding of intricacies that exist between individualizing very extremely a solution to an emergency and having a down-to-earth, practical, rational, and pragmatic control of a dire situation. Though a biopolitical, cum, structuralist inquiry, the analytics of this chapter, as earlier suggested, will in no small measure dovetail into moments of self-examination, as argued by J. Hillis Miller, because a text already contains the operation of self-deconstruction, in which two contradictory principles or lines of argument confront one another but that this undecidability "is always thematized in the text itself in form of metalinguistic statements. In other words, the text does not just contain or perform a self-deconstruction but is *about* self-deconstruction so that a deconstructive reading is an interpretation of the text, an analysis of what it says or means.

(Culler, 2001, p. 17) (italics not mine)

Obviously, this chapter, after all analysis has been done, will announce, to some agreeable extent, that the "text", is, in the present case, a conglomeration of the responses of the Trump government, in statements and deeds, to the coronavirus pandemic, the biopower and structuralism-deconstruction nexus in the interpretive process. The metalinguistic presence in the responses is quite revealing, very unmistakably compelling in the cross-communication between medicine, politics, and ideology. The self-deconstructive trajectory is constructed in the composite picture of the campaign of lies and contradictory statements that trails or is concomitant with the president's responses, something akin to the "continual generating and violating of expectations, a complex interplay of the regular and the random, norms and deviations, routinized patterns and dramatic defamiliarizations" earlier adverted to.

Gerard Gennete's temporality-inclined "five central categories of narrative analysis" will be the starting point for this structuralist elucidation of the politicization of a medical woe of the Covid-19 dimension, as the categories, which will shed light on the chronology of the president's responses, are necessary as a forerunner to building a clear-cut structuralist view of the friction-laden platform of the president's riling against conventionalism in dealing with a demanding issue. In this regard, the *histoire*, which is the sequence in which those events "actually" occurred, will be a structuralist guide to discerning how the responses really panned out. The post "Timeline of Trump's Coronavirus Responses" (*Blog Post*, 2 March2022) serves as a guide for this phase of the structuralism-inspired biopower exegesis. This timeline begins in May 2018, when the Trump administration disbanded the White House pandemic team. In Gerard Gennete's structuralist sensibility, this disbandment of 2018 constitutes both a prolepsis (anticipation) and an analepsis (flashback) or anachrony, both of which would resonate as the conflict between the President and the emergency develops. As a matter of fact, the first case of the pandemic was reported in Wuhan, China, on the 31st of December 2019, about one and a half years after the disbandment. The proleptic preface of the disbandment seems to be a prevision of the cataclysm that will envelop the American political and health institutions as the pandemic sweeps through the country, its terrifying trajectory a history of fatalities and political-ideological controversies. Another event in the *histoire* phase that anticipates the tragedy to come is that the Center for Disease Control (CDC) epidemiologist embedded in China's disease control agency left the post, and the Trump administration eliminated the role. This happened in July 2019, about six months after the first reported case of the disease in Wuhan, China. These two events in America are enough a foreboding of the crisis that would come to settle on America's collective consciousness about mixing politics with the urgency to stop the spread of a deadly pandemic like Covid-19.

The next in the temporality-controlled structuralist configuration of Trump's responses to the pandemic reemphasizes the disaster that awaits the American public. Oblivious to the carnage that the pandemic would cause, Trump observes: "Currently, there are insufficient funding sources designated for the federal government to use in response to a severe influenza pandemic" (*Blog Post*, 2 March 2022). He made this statement in October 2019. The question is, is he anticipating a severe pandemic in the shape of Covid-19 that would be his albatross for the remainder of his presidency? This is because the first confirmed case of Covid-19 in the USA was reported on 21 January 2020. A day afterwards, January 22, Trump is optimistic, whether genuine or feigned, in his belief that "[w]e have it totally under control. It's one person coming in from China. It's going to be just fine" (*Blog Post*, 2 March 2022). The gathering storm is becoming more palpable with each statement or action from the president, and it revs up the anticipatory feeling of the responses, which is suggestive of the Covid-19 debacle developing the exposition stage of a plot in literature. This anticipatory postulation of Genette as part of the "time-order" in the "order" aspect of Trump's responses is reinforced in Trump praising China's handling of the coronavirus: "China has been working very hard to contain the Coronavirus. The United States greatly appreciates their efforts and transparency. It will all work out well. In particular, on behalf of the American People, I want to thank President Xi!" (*Blog Post*, 2 March 2022). This statement of hope issued by the president on 24 January 2020, three days after the first reported American case, was confirmed.

However, the "anticipation" substance is energized by prognostics of dire dimensions even from within the Trump presidency, which the President seems to disavow presumably due to his anti-conventionalist posture. Two statements from two of his aides manifest this unease. On 28 January 2020, four days afterwards, Trump's National Security advisor said this to him: "This will be the biggest national security threat you face in your presidency. . . . This is going to be the roughest thing you face" (*Blog Post*, 2 March 2022). Robert O' Brien could have been apprised of the looming tragedy that his boss was not yet cognizant of or nonchalant about. Seemingly, the president is not perturbed despite another statement of prophetic proportions emanating from another of his aides, Peter Navarro, his Trade advisor, on 30 January 2020, two days after O' Brien came up with the Covid-19 security threat. The aide, through a memo, tells the President:

> The lack of immune protection or an existing cure or vaccine would leave Americans defenseless in the case of a full-blown coronavirus

outbreak on US soil, . . . This lack of protection elevates the risk of the coronavirus evolving into a full-blown pandemic, imperilling the lives of millions of Americans.

(*Blog Post*, 2 March 2022)

These warnings should be enough of a call to action for Donald Trump, but probably due to his obdurate desire to prove conventional wisdom about the disease a falsity, he does not take the prophylactic steps to deal with the emerging emergency.

The anticipation process of the structuralist conceptualization of Trump's responses to the pandemic wears a demeanour of ferocity going by some of his utterances of hope (between 2 February 2020 and 27 February 2020) in spite of the trepidation-loaded cautionary statements from his aides, which were made directly to the president. These are Mr. Trump's statements in the order of their temporal chronology:

"We pretty much shut it down coming in from China."

"I think the virus is going to be – it's going to be fine."

"Looks like by April, you know in theory when it gets a little warmer, it miraculously goes away."

"The Coronavirus is very much under control in the USA . . . the Stock Market starting to look very good to me!"

"CDC and my Administration are doing a job of handling Coronavirus."

"I think that's a problem that's going to go away . . . They have studied it. They know very much. In fact, we're very close to a vaccine."

"The 15 (cases in the US) within a couple of days is going to be down to close to zero."

"We're going very substantially down, not up."

"Well, we're testing everybody that we need to test. And we're finding very little problem. Very little problem."

"This is a flu. This is like a flu."

"It's going to disappear. One day, it's like a miracle, it will disappear."

(*Blog Post*, 2 March 2022)

What makes the president ooze with confidence despite the pall of darkness hovering over the country and his aides' realistic assessment of the situation beats critical watchers hollow. The president's utterances enliven the "anticipation" structure of the responses. At this point, it is clear that the virus had already had a stranglehold on the country and the "anticipation" stage had begun to disappear, giving way to the deathly reality which many high-reasoning Americans had foreseen and predicted. Meanwhile, the president is incognizant that the events that had been described were a prelude, "anticipation" in structuralist analysis, of the problems to come.

There are many other events in statements and actions that may constitute "anticipation" elements but the ones that have been highlighted are deemed appropriate enough for an understanding of the relationship between the President's immediate reaction to the pandemic and when the pandemic got out of hand.

With the "anticipation" stage already constructed and gradually nearing completion, what comes next is the reality phase, or what may be called the "anticipated" phase of the president's responses, which marks the onset of the odious development of the pandemic in the American health sphere, a consequence of events in the "anticipation" "time-order of the narrative". The "anticipation" phase is short but the reality or "anticipated" phase is a long one, not difficult to understand, but its absurdity leaves no one in doubt about the president's actions in the "anticipation" precursor. The first event in the reality phase, after what may be called the termination of the "anticipation" stage, is a House member accusing the Trump regime of being incompetent in handling the health crisis, which translates to the fact that not everybody is deluded about the danger potentials of the coming ravages of the pandemic. Lloyd Doggett, the member of the House of Representatives in question, during a House hearing, warned about mask and test shortages: "The ineptness with which the Trump Administration approached this problem is not only serious, it can be deadly if not changed in the approach" (*Blog Post*, 2 March 2022). The deadliness of the Trump administration's ineptness is indeed part of the "anticipation" phase if one goes by Doggette's concern, and it is a foretaste of the deadliness that will be the upshot of the "anticipation". Now, it is becoming pellucid that deadliness in the anticipation period, which is a forerunner of the "anticipated" (the present phase), is also interchangeable, one and the same with the deadliness of the "anticipated" *salva veritate*, as will be explained briefly shortly.

The "anticipated" phase, which presumably starts with the Doggette accusation, gathers momentum. Between 27 February 2020, when Doggette issued that warning, and 6 April 2020, the death toll from the pandemic had passed 10,000. That means, while Mr. Trump was busy grandstanding during the "anticipation" phase, Americans had already begun to be devastated by the virus. The "anticipated" phase of the president's responses having begun with the Doggette admonitory message, and continued by wearing a deathly dimension through March 2020 to the beginning of April with 10,000 American deaths, is clothed in a more devastating look: between April 6 and April 11, a five-day interval, 10,000 deaths more were recorded, because on April 11, the American death toll was 20,000. Between 11 April and 15 April 2020 (another five-day interval), another 10,000 deaths had taken place, making it 30,000. This "anticipated" regime of Mr. Trump's responses to Covid-19 leaves Americans so much at the mercy of the emergency that "Trump's term in office saw over 25 million confirmed coronavirus cases in the United States, over 400,000 of which resulted in death" (*Blog Post*, 2 March 2022). If the "anticipation" and the "anticipated" phases of the responses (which have now morphed into a narrative of a sort) produced a disjunction between the resident's reactions to the pandemic and the results to those reactions, the "anachrony" phase, which is an integral aspect of the "order" category of Gennete's narratological analysis, acknowledges a far more disconcerting picture of the debacle, as will be discussed next in this structuralist analysis.

Despite the "anticipation" having culminated, and its consequence, which is called the "anticipated" in this chapter for the purpose of clarity, having started to manifest, the wheels of the "order" slant of Gennete's "five central categories of narrative analysis" grinds on, oiled through "anachrony", another temporal phase of the "order" stage. "Anachrony" refers to discordances between "story" and "plot" (Eagleton, p. 91). Put in a more plausible context, "anachrony' " is the "Discrepancy between the chronological order of events and the order in which they are related in a plot" (*Wordnik*). In these Trump responses (now a narrative), "Discrepancy between the chronological order of events and the order in which they are related in a plot" is explicable in the elements of "anticipation" mixing with those of the "anticipated", the latter being the result or culmination of the former. Normally, the "anticipated" phase should follow the "anticipation" chronologically. However, and as observed in the last line of the last paragraph, a far more unsettling portrait of the president's responses is drawn in the "anachrony" chapter of the narrative. Apparently, the confusion in the president's responses becomes more profound as his muddle-headedness becomes more untrammelled and more befuddling despite the crisis wearing a more tragic dimension. That is, while the pandemic moves from one rung of the tragic ladder to higher rungs of the ladder, the president is persistent in issuing statements that are at odds with the seriousness of the moment.

After the Doggette warning (which is arguably the start of the "anticipated" phase, the dire result of the "anticipation" period), one expected Donald Trump to be cognizant of the dangers that his reckless responses in the "anticipation" phase of the crisis portended. However, the contrary is the response from the president, as he continued to manifest an *en core* attitudinal poise to the disasters in the harvest of deaths and the astronomical rate of Covid-19 infections that were already sweeping through the country. Despite the country being in the silent throes of deaths and infections, Trump is undaunted in evangelizing unserious issues and fallacies. One of them is this: "You take a solid flu vaccine, you don't think that could have an impact, or much of an impact, on corona?" [Trump to health officials who answered "No."] (*Blog Post*, 2 March 2022). That health officials could arguably answer in the negative does not stop Trump from averring that "[a] lot of things are happening, a lot of very exciting things are happening and they're happening very rapidly" (*Blog Post*, 2 March 2022). One wonders about the "exciting" things that are happening when deaths and infections on a large scale are "happening". Again, he asserts, "[i]f we have thousands or hundreds of thousands of people that get better just by, you know, sitting around and even going to work – some of them go to work, but they get better" (*Blog Post*, 2 March 2022). This statement is disquieting because in the midst of the disaster, Trump is engaging in triumphalism, boasting about his government's victory, when loss of lives has begun to be the norm. This spirit of triumphalism inspires him to say:

> The United States . . . has, as of now, only 129 cases . . . and 11 deaths. We are working very hard to keep these numbers as low as possible! . . . I think we're doing a really good job in this country at keeping it down . . . a tremendous job at keeping it down. . . . We have a perfectly coordinated and fine-tuned plan at the White House for our attack on CoronaVirus.
>
> (*Blog Post*, 2 March 2022)

These three utterances were made between March 2 and March 4, but roughly a month later, on April 6, 10,000 Americans died. This is a vintage case of "anticipation" mixing with the "anticipated", a structural flux, which only induces the imagery of grief. To emphasize the gravity of the flux, "The World Health Organization categorizes the coronavirus as a pandemic due to its alarming spread and severity" (*Blog Post*, 2 March 2022), on 11 March 2020, almost a month before 10,000 deaths were recorded on April 6. A well-reasoning president, knowing very well that the USA is the centrepiece of globalization, and, therefore, very vulnerable to any problems associated with global influence, in the light of the WHO pandemic pronouncement, would have acted with utmost concern instead of self-aggrandizing and politicizing the calamity.

The WHO pronouncement about the pandemic nature of Covid-19 marks a turning point in its worldwide spread, and, by extension, in the recognition of the fact that the "anticipated" level of the structure of the president's responses is being invigorated. The invigoration notwithstanding, Mr. Trump is undeterred in putting a brave face on the disaster that is unquestionably more indwelling in the American society than looming as is evident in his contention that "[i]t goes away. . . . It's going away. We want it to go away with very, very few deaths. the vast majority of Americans, the risk is very, very low" (*Blog Post*, 2 March 2022), the very day (11 March 2020) WHO recognized Covid-19 as a disease of pandemic proportions. As the ravages continue, the president's responses become more disappointing, and the "anticipated" aftermath to the "anticipation" stage continues to assume disturbing fluxes.

A distinguishable moment in the "anticipated" phase is the statement of self-guilt of the most prominent member of the presidency that is concerned with controlling the disease, Dr. Anthony Fauci, director of the National Institute of Allergy and Infectious Diseases, to Congress, who owned up to the fact that "[t]he system is not really geared to what we need right now . . . That is a failing. Let's admit it" (*Blog Post*, 2 March 2022). Being apolitical to the crisis at hand, Fauci is frank and candid about the insufficiency of the materials needed to stop the rot that is the pandemic overwhelming the nation, admitting that it is a failing on the part of the Trump government. Contrariwise, the president, Donald Trump, is very far from the seriousness that Anthony Fauci is attaching to the crisis. The very day, 12 March 2020, that Fauci admitted the insufficiency of equipment desired to check the pandemic, Trump upped the ante of the "anticipation"-"anticipated" flux with this submission: "You know, you see what's going on. And so I just wanted that to stop as it pertains to the United States. And that's what we've done. We've stopped it" (*Blog Post*, 2 March 2022). While Fauci is clear-sighted about the Trump government not being adequately equipped to deal with the pandemic at that point in time, his boss, the president, is asserting that the virus has been "stopped". The confusion within government (from these opposite views) has not just crept into the "anticipated" phase due to Trump still being glued to his sentiments of the "anticipation" phase, the antipodal stances of Trump and Fauci have strengthened the dire hands of the "anticipated" outcome (phase) of the "anticipation" period.

Almost unstoppably, the "anticipated" phase consequence of the "anticipation" continues, Trump making himself a clog in his own administration's efforts towards fighting off the pandemic. As the situation worsens, Donald Trump continues to grandstand. He tells the USA on 16 March 2020, "Relax, we're doing great" (*Blog Post*, 2 March 2022), in contradistinction to Dr. Anthony Fauchi's view at the same conference where Trump told America to "relax", who is pessimistic that"[t]he worst is ahead for us, [and that the situation had reached] a "very, very critical point now" (*Blog Post*, 2 March 2022). A day earlier, the president had tweeted this: "This is a very contagious virus. It's incredible. But it's something that we have tremendous control over" (*Blog Post*, 2 March 2022). Quite surprisingly, the president continues to glory in self-deceit despite this gloomy pronouncement on March 12:

> As of March 12, the US has seen 1,323 confirmed cases of Covid-19, the disease stemming from the coronavirus, and 38 deaths, according to the Johns Hopkins tracker. Public health officials, including those in his own administration, now estimate that millions of people may eventually be infected with Covid-19.
>
> (Burns, 2020, *Vox*)

Reflecting the intra-administration antagonism that filliped the "anticipated" part of the structure of the responses, public health officials, as read in the just quoted statement, predicted the Covid-19 calamitous infections, but Trump lingers in his "anticipation" behaviours, and the "anticipated" remained aggressively untrammelled, as one can discern in Fauci's support for the position of the health officials: "If we are complacent and don't do really aggressive containment and mitigation, the number could go way up and be involved in many, many millions" (Burns, 2020, *Vox*). Dr. Anthony Fauci is the director of the National Institute of Allergy and Infectious Diseases and a member of the White House coronavirus task force. The warning of Fauci and the public health officials are not after all misplaced. On 3 July 2020, it was announced that Covid-19 cases had reached 539,230,697, and deaths were 6,130,735. (Laughland, 2020, *The Guardian*).

The "anticipated" phase of the president's responses (his responses being the "anticipation") wears an incremental temporal face of sepulchre with the speed with which the number of deaths was rising. In a space of nine days, between 11 April 2020 and 20 April 2020, the country recorded 20,000 deaths. So glum is the death rate that as of 20 January 2021, it became clear that "each day in January, Covid-19 killed an average of 3,100 people in the United States – one every 28 seconds" (*Blog Post*, 2 March 2022). So dreary is the anticipated aftermath of Trump's sorrow-laden reactions in the "anticipation" period that "Trump's term in office saw over 25 million confirmed coronavirus cases in the United States, over 400,000 of which resulted in death" (*Blog Post*, 2 March 2022).

An overview of the "anticipation-anticipated" nexus is provided by a critic who contends revealingly that "Trump is a comorbidity of the COVID-19 pandemic. He isn't solely responsible for America's fiasco, but he is central to it. A pandemic demands the coordinated efforts of dozens of agencies". "In the best circumstances, it's hard to make the bureaucracy move quickly," "It moves if the president stands on a table and says, 'Move quickly.' But it *really* doesn't move if he's sitting at his desk saying it's not a big deal". In the early days of Trump's presidency, many believed that America's institutions would check his excesses. They have, in part, but *Trump has also corrupted them*. The CDC is but his latest victim. On February 25, the agency's respiratory-disease chief, Nancy Messonnier, shocked people by *raising the possibility of school closures and saying that "disruption to everyday life might be severe."* Trump was reportedly enraged. In response, he seems to have benched the entire agency. The CDC led the way in every recent domestic disease outbreak and has been the inspiration and template for public-health agencies around the world. But during the three months when some two million Americans contracted COVID-19 and the death toll topped 100,000, the agency didn't hold a single press conference. Its *detailed guidelines on reopening the country were shelved for a month* while the White House released its own uselessly vague plan (Yong, 2020, *The Atlantic*).

Structuralist Relational Poetics of Saussure, Lotman, Peirce, and Jacobson in Understanding Donald Trump's Covid-19 Presidential Tribulations

Relational dialectics of the structuralist ontology are fundamental to recognizing very distinctly how President Donald Trump dealt with the Covid-19 predicament. These relations, as pointed out in the precursory part of this chapter, are explicable through "parallelism, opposition, inversion, equivalence and so on" (Eagleton, p. 83) as variously established by the literary theorists in the present sub-heading.

Saussurean structuralist ideology identifies with the dualist signification system. Signifying patterns of behavioural manifestations deepen the critical overview of Trump's Covid-19 governing. Trump's double-faced identity is a dire attitudinal construct that encumbers his attempts at taming the pandemic in the United States of America. This two-faced personality is a signpost of a tragic development in the destructive trajectory of the disease. Trump's relationship with China signposts such two-sided attention to the calamitous reality on the ground. In one breath, he chastises World Health Organization about China:

> Had the WHO done its job to get medical experts into China to objectively assess the situation on the ground and to call out China's lack of transparency, the outbreak could have been contained at its source with very little death. . . . Instead, the W.H.O. willingly took China's assurances to [*sic*] face value.
>
> (Ward, 2020, *Politico*)

He strengthens his accusation; responding to a reporter's question about his confidence that the Wuhan Institute of Virology was the origin of Covid-19, Trump is assertive: "Yes, I have. Yes, I have," said the president, without specifying. "And I think the World Health Organization [WHO] should be ashamed of themselves because they're like the public relations agency for China" (*BBC News*, May 2020). He withdrew US funding from WHO because of his allegation that WHO was supporting Chinese denials about the deliberate source of the pandemic. He even attacks the American intelligence community for arguing that Covid-19 "was not manmade or genetically modified" (*BBC News*, May 2020).

In another breath, Trump praised China almost ceaselessly regarding how the country had confronted the outbreak of the disease. Two speeches given here are few testaments to the myriad of plaudits he heaped on China:

> I think China, you know, professionally run in the sense that they have everything under control. . . . I really believe they are going to have it under control fairly soon. You know in April, supposedly, it dies with the hotter weather. And that's a beautiful date to look forward to. But China I can tell you is working very hard.
>
> (Ward, 2020, *Politico*)

Another Trump statement which gave honour to China's anti-Covid-19 struggles is this:

> China seems to be making tremendous progress. Their numbers are way down. . . . I think our relationship with China is good. We just did a big trade deal with China – a very big one. And we've been working

very closely. They've been talking to our people, we've been talking to their people, having to do with the virus.

(Ward, 2020, *Politico*)

These two statements contrasted with the censorious attack on WHO by Trump countenance the signifying parallel between the *langue* and *parole*, between the signifier and the signified. In this exegetic consideration, Donald Trump is the signified, while his speeches are the signifier. His speeches are a sign which makes the curious mind to do some study about the type of personality that the ex-president is with respect to his responses to the pandemic.

The person that Trump is dictates the type of statements that would proceed out of him. This understanding of Trump from the personality down to what he says is in sync with the submission that Saussure "was not interested in what people actually said (parole) but was concerned with the objective structure of signs which made them possible in the first place, and this he called langue" (Eagleton, 2008: 84). Essentially, the personality of Trump as a double-faced person, a double-dealer, leads him to approbate and reprobate in his dealings with personalities and institutions as the pandemic continues its ravaging spread in America. That Trump is also cocooned in political survival more than concern for the public weal is also a signifying revelation in the Covid-19 debacle. Trump contends that "China wanted him to lose his re-election bid in November" (Ward, 2020, *Politico*). This argument creates a signified, a personality with a deep sense of monomania about political victories, to the detriment of developmental values.

The Saussurean dialectics in Trump's behaviour is also apprehended in the ex-president's status leaning in his exhortations to the people about the dangerous potential of the pandemic. The signifying principle in this status manifestation reveals a cleavage between the rich and the poor. The stratified sensibility is a signifying pattern in understanding the behaviour of Donald Trump regarding the effect of the pandemic on the American society. Being a dyed-in-the-wool capitalist, his emotions betray his presidential responsibilities to the people, which should be without deferential reverence to creed, race, and status. As a capitalist, he is the signified of a signifier that is populated by the sensibilities of the rich, which is, to a large extent, an obviation of the sensitivities of the deprived masses. This contradiction in Trump's responsibilities to the people is identified in the divergent information given to the rich and the poor about the parlous nature of the disease, as pointed out in this explanation:

The *New York Times* reports that on February 24, hours before Trump declared on Twitter that the coronavirus was of zero concern and that the stock market was looking hot, senior members of his economic team told wealthy members who sat on the board of the conservative Hoover Institution that things were much more precarious than the President had claimed. Thomas J. Philipson, for instance told the group that he couldn't estimate how badly the virus would affect the American economy, the implication reportedly being that "outbreak could prove worse than . . . [the] Trump administration advisers were signalling in public at the time".

(Levin, 2020, *Vanity Fair*)

Unfortunately, the masses are on the defensive with respect to the political biconsciousness of Donald Trump, a dualist declivity that arises out of a Saussurean sensibility of playing with signification, he a signified of a signifier, which are statements laden with ambivalences which project his stratified glorification of the rich, thereby undermining societal coherence, the poor masses being misinformed about the Covid-19 state of affairs.

Donald Trump's Covid-19 anxieties are critically reflected in the interpretive system of Yuri Lotman's structuralist ideology, in which "meaning only exists contextually, governed by sets of similarities and oppositions" (Eagleton, p. 88), and contiguously reflecting

a system of systems, a relation of relations. It is the most complex form of discourse imaginable, condensing together several systems each of which contains its own tensions, parallelisms, repetitions, and oppositions, and each of which is continually modifying all of the others.

(p. 89)

The Covid-19-combating universe of Trump is not devoid of tensions and anxieties (as can be apprehended from discussions so far) that are characteristic of Lotman's philosophy of structuralism. Lotman's structuralist cosmology, being a relation of relations, appears intractably useful in developing a thesis on the Trumpian mode of containing the pandemic, the psychological, the political, and the economic being systemically connected with the desire to rid the American society of the health emergency, especially in an election year 2020. With these three elements in the crucible of the health debacle, Lotman's concept of tensions and oppositions, are ineluctably priceless in the building blocks of this analysis. The political ante is, therefore, upped, because the American political system is not insensitive to the economic turmoil that is precipitated by a health problem, and this is where the sensibility of Trump is tickled. His allusion to his re-election bid being subverted by China explains the nexus between the politics of survival and controlling the pandemic. The economic relatedness with Trump's tensed-up, stressed, and burdened Covid-19 crusade, as contended earlier, is not far-fetched. A dire warning by a top government official apprises a critic of Lotman's structuralist relational sensibility in the economic consequences of not adequately addressing the growing strength of the disease. Through a memo from Peter Navarro, the Trade advisor to the White House, he starkly "warned Trump administration officials in late January that the coronavirus crisis could cost the United States trillions of dollars and put millions of Americans at risk of illness of death" (Maggi, 2020, *The New York Times*). Navarro emphasizes in his own words:

> The lack of immune protection or an existing cure or vaccine would leave Americans defenceless in the case of a full-blown coronavirus outbreak on US soil. . . . This lack of protection elevates the risk of the coronavirus evolving into a full-blown pandemic, imperilling the lives of millions of Americans.
>
> (Maggi, 2020, *The New York Times*)

The warning from Navarro, given the information coming from China, was unvarnished, as he contended that the "risk of a worst-case pandemic scenario should not be overlooked" (Maggi, 2020, *The New York Times*). His premonition unfortunately came into being on 29 January 2020, when "Mr. Trump was playing down the risks to the United States" (Maggi, 2020, *The New York Times*). Navarro even predicted gloomily that "more than a half-million of Americans could die" (Maggi, 2020, *The New York Times*). His prediction was an understatement, because as of 12 September 2022, 1,044,461 American deaths had been officially recorded, with over 94,973,074 infections (Elflein, 2023, *Statista*). The Trade advisor knows the political deficit in not being pragmatic with truth concerning the situation, and the rest is history, as the pandemic contributed significantly to the death of Donald Trump's re-election aspiration.

The subject of the personality of Mr. Trump additionally inspires an associative contemplation on the dialectics of his Covid-19 hassles. The question is, why did he downplay the minatory aura of the pandemic when it was obvious to him that the disease was wreaking a havoc of fatal dimension? One has to critique Trump's personality and how it impinges on his leadership of the anti-Covid-19 crusade. As immediately explained in the foundational part of this chapter, Trumpism is marked by an unconventionalism that upsets even his own conservative base. This rebellious conservatism creates a Trump that wants to upset the apple cart in the universally prescribed approaches to treating a pandemic, but all to his political peril. This desire to defy conventionalist principles makes him a dauntless navigator of the terrain of behavioural sensitivities, a defiance that has a negative impact on his presidential overseeing of the Covid-19 invasion. Trump rightly evidences an assertion about dauntless individuals, for "[d]*auntless* individuals tend to flout tradition, dislike following routine, sometimes act impulsively and irresponsibly, and are inclined to elaborate on or shade the truth and skirt the law" (Immelman and Griebie, abstract, 2020).

Evidently, in his doughty track of being self-assured, Trump violates the laws guiding safety concerns in controlling the pandemic, his thoughtless and reckless statements and actions militating against world best practices, to the extent that he and his wife, Melania, tested positive for the disease, the peak of a White House endemic of the pandemic. Going about on the campaign trail without using the face mask, which he initially condemned and also mocked his Democrat rival in the 2020 election for wearing it, and not respecting the laws of social and physical distancing, his contracting the disease became a matter of time, putting a lie to his unconventionalism about addressing the contagion. All the political, psychological, and economic issues, including the personal life of Trump, importantly give potency to Lotman's idea that externalities are necessary to developing the internal workings of a thesis, and this intertextual reasoning has invigorated the structuralist analytical space of the main subject of Covid-19 during the Trump presidency.

C. S. Peirce's semiotic establishment of the universe of structuralism has a strong grip over Donald Trump's presidential construction of the Covid-19 universe. The structuralist's triadic signifying postulations of the iconic, the indexical, and the symbolic are verifiably applicable in cognizing the more the structural declivities of the Trump anti-pandemic regime. Peirce's "iconic" representation ("where the sign somehow resembled what it stood for (a photograph of a person, for example") in Trump's supervision of the American anti-coronavirus war identifies parallels between Donald Trump as the president of the country and Trump as the chief supervisor of the campaign to rid the society of the emergency. This, of course, points to Pierce's denotative sense of meaning. As the person in charge of the country's affairs long before the pandemic emerged, the ex-president, Trump, was a picture of crisis after crisis, one of which is the Ukraine scandal, which involved the ex-president coercing Ukraine and some other countries into providing damaging narratives about his co-presidential contestant, Joe Biden, in order to damage the latter's elective prospects. Trump's misinformation about the Russian interference in the American election of 2016, his many issues with women, the 6th January insurrection at the Capitol, the FBI search of his Mar-a Lago residence, which revealed another ungainly uniqueness of his presidency, and other scandal-igniting crises are "iconic" parallels of the crisis that he mothered in his Covid-19 administering. Therefore, pre-Covid-19, Mr. Trump was a cauldron of controversies; his Covid-19 regime was also a minefield of crises, essentially reflecting Pierce's "iconic" structuralist parallel paradigm.

Pierce's second type of sign, the "indexical" structuralist signifying hue, one which indicates that the sign is somehow associated with what it is a sign of, is appreciably existent in Trump's coronavirus escapade. The confusion and pandemonium that are characteristic of Donald Trump's supervision of the Covid-19 challenge are associated, first and foremost, with his chequered private life, his private life a litany of troubles and marital mishaps. One may discern the connotative interpretation in this relationship. One of his classmates, Paul Onish, talks about his rebellious character, as he recalls that he is always getting into trouble "talking out of turn during class, passing notes and throwing spitballs" (*GQ*, 2017), actions which prompted his parents to send him to a strict military academy. Trump owns up to being a deviant in his book, *Art of the Deal*: "As an adolescent, I was mostly interested in creating mischief" (*GQ*, 2017). It is, of course, not surprising when he admitted that he was downplaying the threat of the pandemic, which he did to reassure panic-stricken Americans and an economy in jitters. Unfortunately, Americans, due to the reassuring downplaying of the problem by Trump, treated it with frivolity, and a bad situation got out of hand. By extension, Trump's trouble-laden and chaotic management of the anti-coronavirus regime is a bequest and a signifying progeny, by Pierce's postulate of association, of his troublesome and mischief-loaded private life. He simply superimposes his natural desire for disorder on the Covid-19 issue. The anarchy and turbulence in his marital life and financial dealings, which made him file for bankruptcy over some of his properties (the cause of his delisting from Forbes 100 list) (*GQ*, 2017), are previsions and signifying manifestations of his poorly handled anti-Covid-19 campaign.

At the level of Pierce's "symbolic" sign system, which is akin to Saussure's identifying an arbitrary relationship between a sign and its referent, Trump's coronavirus superintendence may be portrayed as an arbitrary representation of some ideals. The symbolic sign structure may be identified with the "syntagmatic" meaning system (where signs are coupled together with each other in a "chain"). Although arbitrary, the administration of Trump's actions against the pandemic may signpost a destruction of democratic values in the USA due to the ex-president's adversarial attitude to even those that mattered in the control of the deadly virus, his epileptic responses, and his high politicization of an inherently medical emergency. Although not immediately connected with the global standing of a nation, the chaotic nature of facing up to the emergency may be denigrative to the standing of the USA in the committee of nations, for smaller and less significant countries (Nigeria, for instance) were able to contain its spread more effectively than the USA.

In the light of Roman Jacobson's idea of the "poetic" in the analysis of language to explain the peculiarities of a person and the theorist's six communication elements in constructing discourse or a communication space, the course of the pandemic in Donald Trump's America is amenable to the structuralist critical evaluation. The language used by Donald Trump in his attempt to rid the American society of the pandemic leads one to understand his behavioural life and how it impinges on his presidential oversight functions during the pandemic. There are many statements from him as the pandemic rages, but some very instructive ones will be critiqued in order to create a nexus between his personality and his struggles over the emergency. A very illuminating utterance from the ex-president during the pandemic is cognition of his materialist reasoning even when the lives of the citizens were in the throes of a deadly invader. Read him:

China seems to be making tremendous progress. Their numbers are way down. . . . I think our relationship with China is good. We just did a big trade deal with China – a very big one. And we've been working very closely. They've been talking to our people, we've been talking to their people, having to do with the virus.

(Ward, 2020, *Politico*)

Without equivocation, the business at hand when this speech was made was the passion to weaken the grip of the pandemic. However, the enthusiasm of Trump for financial deals, he being impassioned with deal making, seems to overwhelm him even when all thoughts should be about stopping the problem in its strides. He, therefore, expresses and carries too far the mercantilist and rugged mentality of the capitalist ego, thereby reminding people about his unconventionalist proclivity to issues. As a result, he may be construed as a metaphor of ideological extremism. At the associative level, he is realized as a metonymic element in the world of leaders with ingrained class mentality. This statement also shows Trump's inclination to divagate, digress, and, of course, tergiversate between sentences, thereby creating a hermeneutic confusion as to what is really important in a particular situation. This syntactic instability or haziness affects negatively his anti-coronavirus supervision. Another important statement which is a composite representative of all Trump's adversarial confrontations with health professionals during the pandemic is this: "Sporadic for you, but not sporadic for a lot of other people" (Trump's response to a nurse telling him that equipment supply has been "sporadic") (*Blog Post*, 2 March 2022). This riposte from him may signify his distaste for antagonistic views, his presumptuous disregard for any position that rivals his triumphalism in any confrontation or on any issue.

As the pandemic worsened in America, and Trump became more and more confrontational about particularly the need to shut down businesses and keep people at home, he scowled: "WE CANNOT LET THE CURE BE WORSE THAN THE PROBLEM ITSELF" (Haberman and Sanger, 2020, *New York Times*), he being more concerned with the economic challenges of the lockdown than the spread of the virus. The words "cure" and "problem", when understood in the context of the speaker's personality in relation to his pandemic troubles, foreground the ambivalence and paradox that drive his campaign. By juxtaposing the two antithetical words, he problematizes how one is to assess his control over the virus. The trajectory of his struggling for a "cure" is laced with contradictions, which is even more of a problem than his curative reasoning, his suggestion that an unapproved drug could be used to remediate the emergency being a controversial instance. Many statements from Trump may suffice for this analysis but these few can be taken to be typical and characteristic of others not discussed.

Jacobson's structuralist obsession with six elements of communication, viz. "an addresser, an addressee, a message passed between them, a shared code which makes that message intelligible, a 'contact' or physical medium of communication, and a 'context' to which the message refers" makes analysing the Trump novel coronavirus affair an interesting undertaking because of the ex-president's natural tendency towards confusion and his stratified economic model of class distinction. This reminder is necessary: not all six elements are important in specific contexts. However, the addresser, addressee, the message, and the context provide ample opportunity for more clear-sightedness about the reason for the suggested failure of Trump's anti-novel coronavirus presidential journey. As discussed earlier in this chapter, his administration differentiates between the other people and the rich in trying to check the rage of the virus. The diagrams herein underline how Jacobson's structuralist reasoning helps to reveal the bias that is symptomatic of the Trump administration's concern for Americans' Covid-19 plight.

<u>Diagram A</u>

(Addresser) Donald Trump

(Addressee) Americans

Message (Covid-19 has been shot down)

Context (Mar-a-Lago).

In this diagram, Trump addresses the American public. Americans are naturally wont to believe their president. Therefore, they seem to believe his message that the threat of the disease was nil. That the president made this statement in his Mar-a-Lago residence to a journalist is a clear testament that he wanted the message broadcast on a wide scale to Americans. The plan worked but with a grievous consequence: ever-increasing American deaths and infections.

<u>Diagram B</u>

Addresser (Senior members of Trump's economic team)

Addressee (Wealthy and powerful members who sat on the board of the conservative Hoover Institution)

Message (Things were much more precarious than the president had claimed)

Context (Hoover Institution)

The second diagram is the opposite of the first in all its ramifications. Here, sensibility towards status is arguable. Unlike the first, the secretiveness of the message is undisputed because of its political and socially stratified nature. Because of its privatist-public quality, the addresser is different from the first. The addresser is not the president but some members of his economic team, since the message to be delivered should presumably not proceed from the president so as to conceal its partiality because of sensitivity to financial status, a suggestion that a category of people is of more relevance to the administration than the other. The addressee is the wealthy and powerful members of the conservative Hoover Institution. The social difference in the people being addressed is doubtlessly unmistakable. The addressee here constitutes some of the powerful few in the American economic clime, and so, from the administration's prejudiced conscience, seemingly deserves to be more protected. The message to them: the pandemic is more dangerous than Trump asserted, so, take cover. The contest is also ominous, the base of the addressee, Hoover Institution, which reinforces the prejudicial function of the message: tell it to them secretly publicly. This governmental paradox in Trump's governance over the pandemic brings to the fore his scattergun approach to attending to crucial issues.

Northrop Frye's Hero Conceptualization as Constructed in Trump's Responses to the Covid-19 Pandemic

Donald Trump's responses to the pandemic are appreciable in the light of Northrop Frye's hero structuralist conceptualization. This is possible due to Trump's arrogant desire to prevail in every conflict situation, no matter his degree of guilt. The president always sees himself as the hero on any issue and will like to bully himself into relevance and recognition even when it is absolutely unnecessary. The coronavirus pandemic presents critics with another opportune period to observe the president in his hero-sensitive elements. In the battle to defeat the virus, which Trump takes to be an imagined personality war between his ego and the urgency to undermine it, the hero-sensitivity of the president manifests Frye's fictional classification from the hero-making perspective. Frye's assumption that "the hero's power of action, which may be greater than ours, less, or roughly the same" (Frye, 1957: 33), has a grip over Trump's attitude as the pandemic tightened its grip over the American clime. Trump, despite the pall of Covid-19 darkness over the country, continues to play the hero's game, whose power of action, in Frye's structuralist reasoning, he (Trump) considers greater than that of the rest of the country, the result of his presumptuous bearing over the American political system, at least for that moment, because he will later experience the reverse. But in the glory of *hamartia*, his power of action is taken to be greater than that of the rest, and this he exudes through some statements. One such statement is this: "You are not going to die from this pill. . . . I really think it's a great thing to try" (Trump promoting Hydroxychloroquine, not FDA approved to treat coronavirus) (*Blog Post*, 2 March 2022). The president confirms his belief in the drug herein: "I happen to be taking it. . . . A lot of good things have come out. You'd be surprised at how many people are taking it, especially the front-line workers (Beckley and Breuninger, 2020, *CNBC*).

In spite of the drug lacking certification, Trump is urging Americans to take it to counter Covid-19, using his presidential leverage to suggest that his own power of action, power of reasoning, is greater than that of even the Food and Drug Administration (FDA), which did not approve the drug to treat Covid-19. Yet in another instance of Trump showing how his power of action can preponderate over that of others, Trump, in a rhetorical question, suggests a layman's erroneous prophylactic nexus between flu and Covid-19: "You take a solid flu vaccine, you don't think that could have an impact, or much of an impact, on corona?" (Trump to health officials who answered "No") (*Blog Post*, 2 March 2022). Though the health officials answered in the negative (NO), Donald Trump had already shown his power of action by his pseudo-recommendation. The next Trump utterance about the pandemic is unquestionably a classic about who owns the "power of action" in the American political context of the Trump presidency. Regarding the troubled fate of the *Grand Princess* ship, which was stuck and stranded off San Francisco, Trump submitted:

> They would like to have the people come off. I'd rather have the people stay [on the ship]. But I'd go with them. I told them to make the final decision. I would rather – because I like the numbers being where they are. I don't need to have the numbers double because of one ship that wasn't our fault.
>
> (Rostan, 2020, *Market Watch*)

Trump admits that though he differed, he allowed stakeholders, especially in the health sector, who wanted the 3500 on board to disembark, prevail. That he says that he "told them to make the final decision" despite his opposition to the idea implies where the "power of action" is in that situation. Interpreted, if he did not tell them to make the final decision, his negative interest would have prevailed. The most palpable picture of Trump's "power of action" being considered greater than that of not just the rest of America but the rest of the world is cut in Trump's grandstanding and self-hugging about the pandemic nature of Covid-19. The president boasts: "I felt like it was a pandemic long before it was called a pandemic" (*Blog Post*, 2 March 2022). This statement is dismissible because long before and even after the World Health Organization discerned the pandemic force of the disease, Trump's attitude towards it, as is reflected in both the "anticipation" and "anticipated" stages of his responses, was a combination of showboating, insouciance, and, at best, half-hearted commitment to confronting the pandemic. If Trump's bigger-than-thou presumptuousness about the pandemic power of Covid-19 is the most intriguing of his "power of action" being greater than that of the rest, his assertion that "I intended 'to always play it down' [Trump in a private taped interview with Bob Woodward, made public on September 9]" (*Blog Post*, 2 March 2022) can be described as the most flagrant case of abuse of presidential power in order to show that his "power of action" over others' is incontestable, since he knows that his action or his "power of action", more than other people's "power of action", will always determine the success of the fight against the spread of the virus. This of course may have explained his unconventional conservatism as he trivializes and pedestrianizes a deadly and invasive contagion.

It will be appropriate to say that in the context of Trump being at the helm of affairs, when he believes that his "power of action" is greater than that of others, he is, in tragic mode, in a state of hubris, a state of pride, delighting in overweening self-confidence, which makes the hero, that he believes he is, to disregard some moral laws. That said, Frye's "power of action" postulate, as a reminder, also takes into account how the hero's power of action may be lesser than that of the rest, the rest in this regard are health officials and Americans who feel disillusioned by the president's lackadaisical responses to the Covid-19 afflictive incursion. Against the backdrop of this contrariety, Donald Trump seems to be on the defensive, because his "power of action" as the plot of the pandemic unfolds shrinks, becoming lesser than that of his adversaries on the subject. This comparative negativity is announced immediately in the astronomical number of fatalities and infections, and remotely in the failed attempt of Trump to be re-elected due substantially to his failure to come to grips with the seriousness that the diseased situation demanded, for it was reported that "Former president Donald Trump lost the 2020 election largely because of his handling of the coronavirus pandemic, according to a post-election completed by Trump campaign pollster Tony Fabrizio" (Dawsey, 2021, *Washington Post*), although he still trumpets the lie that he won the election.

That his responses to the pandemic were his Achilles heels in his failed bid to be returned as the president underlines ultimately that his "power of action", at the risk of being rehashed, was lower than that of adversarial individuals and entities, making it crystal clear that he was less than the hero that he was in the crisis as far as Northrop Frye's hero's power of action postulation is concerned. In Freud's second version of the topographical psychoanalytic argumentation (Wright, 1998: 10), that Trump's "power of action" was less than that of his responses-to-the-pandemic represents the "superego", a (. . . representative of parental and social influences upon the "drives", a transformation of them rather than an external agency). These influences act as subversive forces to the initial Trump's triumph, when his "power of action" prevailed over that of the rest, which can be called his "id". This "id" is "a term applied retrospectively to the instinctual drives that spring from the continual needs of the body" (p. 10). Without equivocation, the needs of the body of Donald Trump border on the need to predominate in any argumentative ambience.

Donald Trump's Covid-19 Debacle Against the Backdrop of Frye's Narrative Categories

The "four narrative categories" of "the comic, romantic, tragic and ironic" (Eagleton, p. 80) in Northrop Frye's criticism of the structure of the narrative can also engage one's knowledge of how Donald Trump takes on the destructive presence of Covid-19 in the American socio-political quagmire. It has to be restated that though these four categories are, in Frye's view, a staging ground for literary criticism, they can be a path to understanding a non-literary phenomenon; after all, the non-literary narrative may be of like structural build with its literary equivalent, and it (the non-literary narrative) can have the same structuration with the literary prose, as will be comprehended presently. According to Frye, "The theme of the comic is the integration of society, which usually takes the form of incorporating a central character into it" (Frye, 1957: 43). Contrarily, the central character in the Covid-19 conversation of the American society, Donald Trump, seems not interested in the integrative discourse because the more the pandemic assumed a deathly dimension, the farther the president was from his people, as is explicable in his actions and inactions that have been dissected earlier in this chapter. This anti-integrative situation is replicated in the analysis of the ironic narrative category of Frye's postulation.

There are two modes of reasoning out irony in Trump's understanding of the medical emergency. In the first instance, Trump instantiates the pseudo-reverse of Frye's tragic irony, wherein the "hero does not necessarily have any tragic hamartia or pathetic obsession: he is only somebody who gets isolated from the society. Thus, the central principle of tragic irony is that whatever exceptional happens to the hero should be utterly out of line with his character" (Frye, p. 41). This pseudo manifestation of Trump in Frye's connotation of tragic irony is an emblem of his ambivalent character in many crucial situations – he a symbol of prevarication for survival. This ambivalence now presents itself in an adverse position to Frye's tragic irony, where he has a "tragic hamartia or pathetic obsession" (p. 41) but at the same time "gets isolated from the society" (p. 41). Trump's pseudo-phenomenon is made bolder in that his re-election bid ends in tragedy, but his tragic course is utterly within his character, the fount or source of his "tragic hamartia or pathetic obsession".

Trump is isolated from the society on account of his arrogance about power and his passion to be distinct, which makes him to discountenance veritable concerns about the pandemic. In the second instance of Frye's ironic construction that is identifiable in Trump's presidential communication with the pandemic is the "*pharmakos* or scapegoat" (p. 41) character frame. To Frye, the "*phamarkos* is neither innocent nor guilty" (p. 41). The issue is that Trump's re-election prospects were dampened and destroyed by the outbreak of the pandemic, which impinged negatively on the American economy, a vital success factor in any American election. Unfortunately, the pandemic was not of his making; he just became a scapegoat of adventitiousness or accident of circumstance. Therefore, Donald Trump's innocence is established in the light of the accidental nature of the Covid-19 outbreak. However, his guilt is proven in the politics of individualism, recklessness, and insouciance that he introduced into controlling the plague. He allowed his anti-establishment beliefs to get the better part of him, and the rest is history.

Frye's romantic narrative category has an eloquent presence in the former president's romanticization of extreme Republicanism, which affected his approach to solving the problem. Trump's overly expressiveness about Republicanism is a reflection of Frye's part-conceptualization of romance as being "characterized by the acceptance of pity and fear, which in ordinary life relate to pain, as forms of pleasure; It turns fear at a distance, or terror, into the adventurous; fear at contact, or horror, into the marvellous" (p. 37). Actually, as President Trump romanticizes an extreme sense of conservatism in his attitudinal concern for the pandemic, he builds a paradoxical complex of sympathy and dread by taking some steps towards addressing the emergency, but at the same time, in the spirit of Frye's romance, he turns the pains in the tragedy into a sybaritic (pleasure-seeking) satisfying of his anti-conventionalism. He derives so much pleasure from the tragic turn of events that he approbates and reprobates about checking the spread of the disease, issuing statements that smack of frivolity like "This is a very contagious virus. It's incredible. But it's something that we have tremendous control over" (*Blog Post*, 2 March 2022). Contrarily, the numbers of deaths and infections continue to rise exponentially so terribly that on 26 March 2020, "[t]he United States becomes the country with the most confirmed coronavirus cases. A title it keeps for the remainder of Trump's time in office" (*Blog Post*, 2 March 2022).

At a point, the former president lapses into political adventurousness, a revealing part of his negligent watch over the scourge. A statement like "I intended 'to always play it down' " (*Blog Post*, 2 March 2022) underscores the laxity with which he conducted affairs about the plague. This adventurousness becomes more intense when he castigated members of the Democratic opposition in trifling manners despite the deathly plot that was in the air. He is antagonistically derisive of one of them:

> We've had a big problem with the young, a woman governor from – you know who I'm talking about – from Michigan . . . I love Michigan, one of the reasons we are doing such a GREAT job for them during this horrible Pandemic. Yet your Governor, Gretchen "Half" Whitmer is way in over her head, she doesn't have a clue. Likes blaming everyone for her own ineptitude!
>
> (*Blog Post*, 2 March 2022)

Another Democrat is also a subject of his scurrilous attacks: "We're doing a great job for the state of Washington and I think the Governor . . . he's constantly chirping and I guess complaining would be a nice way of saying it" (*Blog Post*, 2 March 2022). All this rash brinkmanship, an adventure into the politics of emotionality by an extremely politically sensitive Trump, undermines the solemnity of the emotional outpouring that is concomitant with the situation.

For the sake of emphasis, all Trump's actions, inactivity, and passivity that subverted his anti-Covid-19 struggles are, as a reminder, a subject of deconstruction in this chapter, because they have been subjected to serious scrutiny about morality and ideological sensibilities, in the process announcing their dysfunctionality for developmental prospects.

The Nigerian Socio-Political Ambience in the Light of Donald Trump's Response to the Coronavirus Pandemic

The Nigerian state defines itself very vividly as an empathy with the totalitarian blueprints of necropolitics and structural chaos due to decades of lawlessness, misrule, and political waywardness, all of which contribute negatively to environmental peace. Environmental degradation is caused partly by poverty and war of any shape, and to a large extent, these are aftermaths of the elements of structural chaos and biopower narcissism pointed out earlier. This picture of a retrograde identity attracts a similitude with Donald Trump's consciousness of the pandemic, his obsession with political preponderance and personality supremacy being symptomatic of the governmental maladies that plague the Nigerian nation. Analysing the Trump pandemic affair from the biopower-structuralist viewpoint, the behavioural confluence above being of the essence, one is able to discern some implications of Trump's Covid-19 indiscretions for the Nigerian polity. In the light of the primary focus of this exegetic exercise being on ex-president Trump's mishandling of the pandemic, the Nigerian equivalent will, as earlier asserted, be explored minimally. This discussion of these implications will straddle the socio-environmental, economic, political, and even educational facets of the Nigerian governmental system.

In the first place, one must note that the Nigerian administration of the Covid-19 pandemic was not, surprisingly though, as chaotic as that of the engagement under the presidency of Donald Trump. What does this imply?: a destruction of the myth of superiority of the advanced democracies of the world over a country with the nascent democratic feeling, a contradistinction that buries the oft-believed conception that ugly things only happen in the Third World environment. While Trump was busy engaging in political gymnastics and interpersonal squabbles, the Nigerian government, maybe conscious of its developing nation status and the consequence of allowing the problem to get out of hand, was forthright in embracing the seriousness that the pandemic deserved. All hands were on deck, from the centre to the constituent units, all collaborating effectively to deny the pandemic an American-style foothold in the society. Another relevance of the Trump Covid-19 misery for Nigeria is the exhortation to powers-that-be that people should be the centrepiece of government's administrative concerns, and not the ego of the leaders or administrators, as was the paradigm in Trump's America.

However, the egocentric mien of the leader proves to be a frailty in the Nigerian system in some isolated cases of the management of the pandemic. Nigeria being a country of a conglomeration of unpredictable politicians was not insulated from the Trumpian unconventional syndrome, implying very gravely that there can be similitude in the leaning towards developmental blunders through either some sense of self-absorption or suspicions about the Nigerian corruption problem, or both. Some politicians were suspicious of the campaign of the National Centre for Disease Control (NCDC) to stop the spread of the disease, for they argued that the body was being more vociferous than the gravity of the problem demanded, so as to attract more financing from the government. The governor of Kogi State, Mr. Yahaya Bello, could have been propelled by either self-absorption or corruption in his response to the Covid-19 problem in his state. He was, therefore, fervently averse to the popular view that the virus was in every Nigerian State. In order to justify his nil-position, he made false claims of mass testing in Kogi State. He stated thus:

After one month of intensive testing by their workers and officials, not one single person tested positive. The NCDC, ministry of health and my state incident management team went around. They went to institutions, market places, motor parks, streets, villages, towns and cities and not one single individual was confirmed positive. When students are resuming schools, we carry out tests on both indigenes and non-indigenes, indidebes [sic] and there has never been one single positive test. We have NYSC camp in Kogi and we have received three to four batches. The NCDC, NYSC officials and the military with our incident management team tested all the CORP members. Every stream comprises of about 700 to 750 persons and nobody tested positive.

(Onyeji, 2020, *PremiumTimes*)

His statement was far from the truth because "Kogi, a state of almost 3.5 million people, had tested only 425 samples by December 11, the national situational report published December 12 by the NCDC showed" (Onyeji, 2020, *PremiumTimes*). Governor Bello is vigorous in arguing that "in Kogi, we say we have no COVID-19 and actually as a matter of fact, we have no COVID-19" (Onyeji, 2020, *PremiumTimes*). His stance is not far from Trump's querulous position, both contesting the medically incontestable. The relevance of Trump's *faux pas* for the Nigerian Covid-19 context, respecting Governor Bello's resistance to tests, reinforces the existing fear by some people of the politicization of the scourge, the fear of the vaccine itself, and the fear of some governmental officials (in the Nigerian case) turning the pandemic into a cash cow of corruption. The politicization of the scourge is a veritable parallel with Trump's American management of the problem.

As fault lines in American democracy are being laid bare through President Trump's chaotic Covid-19 management, some fault lines in the Nigerian socialscape are also baring their degenerate, ugly features, foregrounding deep implications for the growth of Nigeria's desire for a knowledge-based environment and a cohesive society. The Nigerian educational system takes a big hit, the long lockdown necessitating a creative and ICT-inspired reaction. Like the Trump status-inclined passion about communicating with the people, the Nigerian educational decadence reveals itself partly in the uneven development in the country, and this unevenness is especially pronounced in the commercial capital, Lagos State. The resort to off-class, home lessons through the use of the internet became necessary. However, the underprivileged, particularly children in the rural places, seemed highly disadvantaged because of their poverty-induced inaccessibility to the vitals of the internet age. Despite the state government providing radio and TV lessons, the reality is bleak for poor "families that earn below \$1 per day and faced harsh economic realities due to the four-week lockdown in the state, [as] the purchase of radios or TV might be a trade-off that they cannot afford" (Amorighoye, 2020, *World Economic Forum*). The ICT angle is more precarious for these rural, poor students because

[t]he COVID-19 pandemic is revolutionizing digital and online education globally but kids in rural and underserved communities in Lagos State, Nigeria, are being left behind as they are not equipped to adapt or transition to the new methods of learning.

(Amorighoye, 2020, *World Economic Forum*)

If the poor students found it hard to buy radios and TVs, one wonders how extremely difficult it would be for them to access more expensive and more complex-to-learn ICT equipment in order to take off-person lessons from home, the upshot of a system that glorifies the stratified consciousness, a biased consciousness that partly underlines the unravelling of the Trump administration's inclining towards keeping the rage of Covid-19 in check.

The Nigerian social sphere, like the American Covid-19 debacle under President Trump, also spectacularly explains itself through a sordid timeline, a chronology of events that announces the ineptitude and general laxity that assails government's ability to tackle a problem with grave environmental fallouts because of its attendant and growing threat to social life and security. An environmental epidemic rears its ugly head; so epidemic it is that an epidemic of sorrows, tears, diseases, and frustration becomes its direct and indirect results. Although the Nigerian subject at issue predates Trump's pandemic travails, the emotional blunders committed by the governing actors in the two issues create a nexus in the world of Gennette's postulation about "prolepsis (anticipation) and analepsis (flashback) or anachrony". The response of the Nigerian government to the epidemic of criminal abductions in the Nigerian polity seems to parallel the responses of Trump to the pandemic in the USA. Like the Trump case, the Nigerian government's reasoning about "anticipation" and analepsis (the past) seems jaundiced and error-prone, as will be revealed anon in some sort of Nigerian timeline about some criminal, ransom-induced abductions. It has to be reemphasized that abductions ignite environmental deterioration in various forms: penury, lack of productivity due to attacks on farmers, disease, environmental pillaging as a result of violent exchanges between non-state actors and the military, frustration, and an overall sense of psychological degeneration.

The abductions, which seem to be endless, are so ferocious that deaths and trauma are left in their trails. The abductors particularly go for a section of the vulnerable segments of the human population: students in schools. Unfortunately, a timeline of some of these abductions reprises the governmental indecencies that are the bane of Trump's coronavirus travails, a situation where the Nigerian government discountenances analepsis (the past) and so its sense of anticipation is diseased. Instead of the government activating its anticipatory feelings by recognizing the warnings about abduction threats, the reverse is demonstrated. The laxity, incompetence, irresponsibility, and arrogance of power that define the timeline of Trump's Covid-19 battles manifest themselves in the timeline of some abduction cases in Nigeria. These cases concern abductions in schools. Between one event of abduction and the other, a tale of confusion seems to be the narrative emerging from the government and its officials. So confusion-brained was the government that it did not know exactly how many students were abducted at Chibok. Aljazeera explains the confusion:

> A day after the April kidnappings, Nigerian authorities claimed that the number of abducted was just over 100 young women, and that most had already been rescued. But that number later rose, and the military was forced to recant its statement and acknowledge that it had not rescued any of the girls.
>
> (Kutsch, 2014, *Aljazeera*)

With the noisome distance between prolepsis (anticipation) and analepsis (past), the reactions of the then president, Goodluck Jonathan, and his wife, Patience Jonathan, bespeak the frivolity that the government was accused of in the wake of the attack. Having not acted in line with the warnings that the abduction was in the offing, the president, or the government becomes culpable when Gennete's structuralist concept of anticipation is considered. The president only found it fit to meet with stakeholders, the school, security, and state officials, two weeks after the kidnapping, when the kidnappers had already begun ruminating on what to do with their "trophy". So comfortable was the Boko Haram leader, Abubakar Shekau, that he revelled in his prize: "I abducted your girls. I will sell them in the market, by Allah" (Kutsch, 2014, *Aljazeera*). Meanwhile, while he was delighting in his criminal victory, the Nigerian government was engrossed and embroiled in silence, inaction, and aimless accusations against anybody that mattered, especially people protesting the abduction. Nigeria's First Lady then, Patience Jonathan, was virulent in this regard, as she "personally intervened against leaders of the protest movement, claiming the demonstrators should be arrested and blame themselves if anything happened to them" (Kutsch, 2014, *Aljazeera*).

Trump's foolhardiness and governmental self-glorification are also a defining malevolent construct in the Nigerian Chibok kidnap saga, as the Nigerian government, out of a spurious feeling of nationalism, wanted no external help in freeing the girls. President Jonathan argued with Mark Simmonds, UK's Africa minister at the time, on 15 May 2014, that "Nigeria's intelligence and military services must solve the ultimate problem" (Mcque, 2017, *The Guardian*). The London *Guardian* reported details about the refusal:

> Notes from meetings between UK and Nigerian officials, obtained through the Freedom of Information Act, also suggest that Nigeria shunned international offers to rescue the girls. While Nigeria welcomed an aid package and assistance from the US, the UK and France in looking for the girls, it viewed any action to be taken against kidnapping as a "national issue". . . . In a mission named Operation Turus, the RAF conducted air reconnaissance over northern Nigeria for several months, following the kidnapping of 276 girls from the town of Chibok in April 2014. "The girls were located in the first few weeks of the RAF mission," a source involved in Operation Turus told the *Observer*. "We offered to rescue them, but the Nigerian government declined."
>
> (Mcque, 2017, *The Guardian*)

The Chibok abduction happened on 14 April 2014. This abduction is a more reprehensible case of disregard for "anticipation" based on "analepsis" (the past). A security-conscious government would have expected an encore of the Chibok-like kidnap, after all Boko Haram had/has not been destroyed; but that was not to be as is evident in the next discussion. The next school abduction (Dapchi School girls' kidnap) took place in the life of another president, Muhammadu Buhari. The Chibok attack would have taught a security-sensitive Nigerian government a lesson in securing its vulnerable citizens, but the Trump governmental ailment of nonchalance was allowed to drive the conversation. The behavioural sequence of the Nigerian government after the first students' abduction invariably strikes a semblance with Trump's inaction. The Dapchi School girls' kidnap of 19 February 2018, almost four years after Chibok, turns out to be another statement in history repeating itself in a sordid manner. The government failed in two respects of the "anticipation"-cum-"analepsis" structuralist reasoning. The government was notified in advance of the threat of the abduction, yet, the criminality did not come unstuck. Secondly, the government was unresponsive to the reality that there could be a repeat of the Chibok episode.

The two kidnap cases highlight, as earlier affirmed, the lack of care that is characteristic of Nigerian governments about the people. From reports, the

Chibok incident, which took place during Jonathan's reign, was a result of revolting unconcern and negligence about the security of the nation. Unfortunately, Jonathan's error about security was not enough of a lesson for his successor, Muhammadu Buhari, as the Dapchi affair was a perfect rehash of the Chibok blunder, as informed by the media:

> At the time Boko Haram kidnapped almost three hundred girls from a school in Chibok in 2014, reports surfaced that the Nigerian security forces had advance intelligence, but that they failed to take the necessary preventive action. In February 2018, Boko Haram kidnapped 110 girls from the Government Girls Science and Technical College at Dapchi in Yobe state. Amnesty International released a report of the February kidnapping, concluding that the Nigerian security forces again ignored advanced warnings of an impending Boko Haram kidnapping operation up to four hours before the attack.
>
> (Campbell, 2018, *Blog Post*)

Although, under immense political pressure, the government was forced to negotiate the release of the Dapchi girls from the den of their Boko Haram captors, the damage to the country's concept of security system had been faulted. The Dapchi blunder due to insensitivity to the norm of "anticipation" notwithstanding, seemingly intractable criminal abductions continue to belie the Nigerian government's readiness to secure the lives of its citizens: the Kankara boys (of Government Science Secondary School, Kankara) (Katsina State) kidnap of 11 December 2020; the Dandume foiled kidnap bid (of 80 students of an Islamic school in Katsina State) of 19 December 2020; the Kagara, Niger State, abduction of 41 students (of Government Science Secondary School) of 17 February 2021; the abduction of 317 female students in Zamfara State, on 26 February 2021; the kidnap of 39 students of Federal College of Forestry Mechanisation, Kaduna State, on 11 March 2021; the kidnap of about 20 students and 2 staff of Greenfield University, Kaduna State, on 20 April 2021; and the abduction of dozens of students from an Islamic school in Niger State, on 30 May 2021, are evidence of the inability of the Nigerian government to stem the tide of what has become a menacing epidemic, a cash cow for criminal elements, who have discovered in the forest a more suitable means of harvesting delinquent, vile, and reprobate rewards, contributing indirectly to deforestation and environmental degradation through continuous dehumanisation of humans in an eco-friendly environment. That the government also lied that it paid ransom for the release of the Dapchi girls implies a gruesome equivalence with the disingenuousness of Donald Trump in taking care of Americans during the pandemic. A UNO report averred,

> Contrary to the report by the Nigerian government through the Minister for Information Lai Mohammed, the government paid a "large ransom" to free scores of female students kidnapped by the Boko Haram

from their school in Dapchi, Yobe State, earlier this year, the United Nations has said.

(Haruna, 2018, *Premium Times*)

A more outrageous aspect of disdain for prolepsis (anticipation) is the report that the then Minister of Education, Mr. Nyesom Wike, warned the then governors of Borno, Adamawa, and Yobe states of the security problem in the states and advised them, through a letter, to relocate students of secondary schools to safe places so that they could do their WASC exams there. Not hearkening to Wike's advice, thereby running "foul" of Gennette's postulate about prolepsis (anticipation), Kashim Shetima, the then governor of Borno State (now the Vice President of Nigeria) disregarded the advice; a month after the directive, on 14 April 2014, Boko Haram terrorists invaded Government Girls Secondary School in Chibok and abducted 276 female students. This implies that, like the Trump Covid-19 affair, the governor might have been prompted to disregard the advice because of egocentric sentiments, since he could not have liked to be dictated to by an "ordinary" minister. So, the anticipated attack took place, much to the chagrin of Nigerians. Wike was livid, and he explained:

WAEC wrote to me to inform me that we have a security problem in that particular school and therefore they wouldn't want exam to take place in that school. I wrote a letter to the governor to say that this is what we have observed, so please there should no be [*sic*] exam in that school, move them to the city and get an alternative place because of the security reports we have. The governor never reverted to me or wrote to me to say we are doing this or we are doing that. We wrote a letter a month to the time, not that we just wrote it within two days.

(*Foundation for Investigative Journalism*, 2022)

The Nigerian environmental landscape, in another regard, is also a victim of governmental lassitude, another reminder of how relevant Trump nonchalance about the Covid-19 pandemic to the Nigerian governmental situation can be. Recently, due to heavy torrential downpours, many towns and cities in Nigeria were submerged in fluvial overflows. These flooded environments are now being subjected to all the indecencies and discomforts that are the upshot of such probably unpredictable occurrences. The most disheartening of the aquatic plot of sorrow is its possible cause, which may be linked to lack of interest in town planning and egregious disregard for warnings about impending natural disasters, which shares similarity with Trump's initial disregard for warnings about the fatal repercussion of his ego-centred concern for the pandemic. This disregard for cautions and exhortations about the imminence of the inevitable menace is explicable in Nigeria's Minister for Water Resources' denial that Lagdo Dam in Cameroun caused Nigeria's floods. Although Mr. Suleiman Adamu said that the Lagdo Dam was not the main cause (as some experts had argued), he admitted that the planned mitigating plan for water from the dam to be arrested was the construction of Dasin Hausa Dam in Adamawa but which "was still on the drawing board" since the early 1990s. A profound interpretation of the non-construction of the Adamawa Dam is that if water from the Lagdo Dam is released, there will be flooding in many Nigerian towns and cities. The dam was not constructed due to governmental irresponsibility.

Very outrageously, the minister, despite admitting that the Dasin Hausa Dam in Adamawa was not in existence as planned, was infertile in his arrogance that "Even this one, they are the ones who should keep us informed about the level of the water but they didn't. They informed us 24 hours after" (Akwueh, 2022, *Voice of Nigeria*). Instead of the minister being frank that the government was absolutely culpable for the floods, he still engaged in the subterfuge of accusing Cameroun of some inaction. Albeit he said that "the flood was due to water flowing from the tributaries of River Katsina Ala and others into River Benue due to heavy downpour" (Akwueh, 2022, *Voice of Nigeria*), it will be difficult to believe his statement in the light of the fact that the Dasin Dam, which should have been used to dam water from Cameroun's Lagdo Dam, was not in place in Nigeria. But for space issues, so much more implications of the Trump Covid-19 episode for the Nigerian socio-political world would have been very expansively explicated.

Donald Trump's Response to the Coronavirus Pandemic: The South African Anti-Covid-19 Social Locus in Perspective

The South African government's response to the Covid-19 pandemic in the light of Mr. Donald Trump's epileptic engagement with the disease can be described as vigorous despite the overwhelming force of the invasion, which has brought into view some particular developing-nation-inspired challenges. The country also has its lows in respect of the anti-development consequences of the pandemic, which are not a result of the non-commitment of leadership, as was the case in America's Trump. The South African paradigm in this chapter is most revealing because "[t]he country has recorded the most coronavirus cases and deaths in Africa, with more than 3.9 million confirmed infections and upwards of 101,000 deaths" (*Aljazeera*, 2022). The government, against the backdrop of this uncomfortable reality, has to contend with myriad problems, but in a subdued manner, its management of the disease can be analysed taking into consideration the disjointed performance of Mr. Donald Trump when he was the president of the United States of America.

The relevance of the Trump status-influenced affectation with the pandemic is understood in the South African stratified consciousness as it affects the rural areas of the country. Dr. Rosie Burton, an MSF infectious diseases specialist, voices her concern about this: "It is another reality in rural South Africa. . . . What the epidemic has done in a place like rural KwaZulu-Natal is expose the horrendous inequity in the health system" (Apo Group, 2020).

That emphasis has been on the urban areas in the struggle to tame the Covid-19 pandemic is no understatement because of the high number of infections in the cities and the importance of the cities in the economic development of a nation. The South African coronavirus experience is invariably not an exception, as "it is increasingly clear that COVID-19 has not been a solely urban public health phenomenon" (Apo Group, 2020). The status-driven consequences are due to the fact that in the rural areas "[t]he distances between clinics are greater, there are fewer health resources and govern- ance systems are often multi-layered, to name just a few of the challenges" (Apo Group, 2020).

The status problem as it affects rural areas is not helped by an egregious lack of enlightenment in the townships regarding the nature of the health emergency. Because of the distance between rural dwellers and information concerning true perspectives about the problem, the concentration on cities being the obsession of government officials, rural dwellers were turned in the opposite direction. A rural leader attests to this influence of lack of facts on the people:

> There were so many rumours when this thing started, because people saw death on the TV. When they were told there would be testing, there were those older ones who thought that the government was coming to *jova* (inject) them with the disease, and they went to hide. In this place, people trust and listen to traditional leaders, and when they are sick many of our people first turn to a traditional healer.
>
> (Apo Group, 2020)

The good side of the rural areas story is the effervescence of the government, non-governmental agencies, and very conscionable and concerned individu- als about the neglect of the hinterland in the anti-Covid-19 crucible. This con- vergence of human agents was a collaborative effort aimed at putting in place an agenda that would save the rural hemisphere the horrors of the pandemic. The activity of the MSF (*Médecins sans frontières*) is noticeable herein for, one of its members, George Mapiye, MSF deputy field coordinator, averred, "We needed to implement prevention measures without delay" (Apo Group, 2020). With "a diverse, multi-sectoral emergency response committee, which met weekly in the first months", an aggressive enlightenment campaign was embarked upon on pension payment days, when thousands of people flock to town, being the body's target, and education on the need to respect restric- tion instructions was made an issue.

Besides the multi-pronged involvement of non-governmental institutions like the MSF, the South African anti-Covid-19 campaign is also gracefully complemented by the volunteering initiatives of altruistic South Africans, who deemed it imperative to take care of societal vulnerables like the old people. These young volunteers, assisted by UNICEF, synergized with Department of Health, Department of Social Development, Boxer Supermarkets (one of the pay-points where pensioners collect their grant), and other implementing partners, to help out the old people in registering for vaccination, since many of these old folks lack the necessary technological know-how that the process entailed (Bagherioromi, 2021, *UNICEF South Africa*).

That leaders of African countries banded together through a high level of collective consciousness in countering the pandemic previsions a less than noxious encounter with the problem, as distinct from and at odds with the Trump-led American government's war against the pandemic. This success of this African united front is proclaimed in this report:

> As COVID-19 infections soar in the United States, the African conti-nent is bracing for a smaller surge, defying predictions that it would be hardest hit. According to Africa's top medical official, that's because the continent behaved as one indivisible unit in fighting the virus, with lead-ers working together to impose lockdowns, enforce mask requirements and work with continental officials to improve testing and treatment. "The key, unifying leadership of the continent very early on in Febru-ary has been a very critical factor in moderating the spread of the virus on the continent," Dr. John Nkengasong, director of the Africa Centers for Disease Control and Prevention, said to a collection of global health experts during a virtual meeting this week. "As a matter of fact, if the continent didn't go into a massive shutdown early on in March, with the rates in South Africa, for example, doubling every two days, I think that would have been a severe pandemic in South Africa."
>
> (*VOA*, 2020)

The American Covid-19 world, especially as governed by Mr. Trump, con-trasted with the African collective sensibility, which images the South African robust approach, is a noisome demonstration of the politicization of a deli-cate life-involving health concern. Dr. Antony Fauci, who heads the National Institute of Allergy and Infectious Diseases, in the country hit hardest by the pandemic, the United States, voices his apprehension over the American's frivolous attitude towards the emergency:

> If those five public health measures [the five steps everyone must take to avoid the respiratory virus: wear a mask; keep a two-meter distance from others; avoid crowds; conduct any gatherings outdoors instead of indoors and regularly wash hands] were adhered to, universally and consistently over the country, it is clear from our previous experience with other nations and even regions in our own country, we would not be having the degree of surging of cases that we are currently seeing.
>
> (*VOA*, 2020)

The American unfavourable attitude to the coronavirus adversity is reflected in the behavioural ambivalence of the country's political leadership, because " [i]n some U.S. states, political leaders have embraced those measures. In others, state governors have contested the importance of masks or declined to impose restrictions they say would hurt businesses" (*VOA*, 2020). Impliedly, the African, nay, South African, instruments of slowing down the desolation of the disease are less personalized, less prejudicial, and less discriminatory than the American path to addressing the scourge, and so highly effectively frontal.

The South African assault on the disease was on that account a reflection of African governments' earnestness about the giving the pandemic a rough ride on the continent. With the first reported case in March of 2020, "a 500 billion rand stimulus was announced in response to the pandemic" (Omarjee and Magubane, 2020, *News24*); the government was, therefore, clear about the perilous nature of the problem and so was determined to address it frontally. The South African Covid-19 challenge, like it happened in some countries, was compounded by the evasive nature of the disease as it continued to create strains of various sorts, thereby giving health authorities more cause for concern. With local cases of the Delta and Alpha variants discovered in the country, the South African Covid-19 environment became very tense, and the government acknowledged that the battle against the pandemic would be a long one, especially with waves after waves of its recrudescence appearing to slow down existing progress. At a juncture, the worrisome complexion of the problem reared its head with the alert raised to level 4 "with the Delta variant fast becoming the dominant strain in the country", and doctors in Johannesburg characterize "the system there as beyond its breaking point, with insufficient beds and barely enough oxygen" (McKenzie, 2021, *CNN*). This was just about 16months into the pandemic.

There is an obvious similarity between the US and South African pandemic contexts because both countries had breaking point experiences in some cities due to different reasons. While the unconventional management of the Covid-19 problem by the former president, Donald Trump, might have been responsible for the American health quagmire, the developing nation status of the South African economy may be the cause of its overwhelmed and overburdened health facilities. Despite its economic lows, the country was still able to replicate the Moderna Covid-19 in February 2022, highlighting the seriousness with which the country was addressing this affliction of extensive dimension.

The fifth wave of Covid-19 in South Africa initially appeared to be very perplexing and troubling in the South African pandemic story as it was inspired by another variant of the disease, known as Omicron. Though the variant had its provenance in Botswana, it was brought to the awareness of World Health Organisation by the South African authorities because of its dangerous potential. Its immediate effects were tough for people in the southern African region. Travel bans for people in that area were implemented by some countries due to the high transmissibility and communicability of the strain; though it was reported that it was less severe than the Delta strain in terms of hospitalization, the high number of hospitalizations remained a cause for apprehension.

The relevance of the story of Omicron in the South African Covid-19 plot, as contrasted with Trump's coronavirus episode, is the celerity with which it was dealt with. Unlike Trump's diseased campaign, the advent of Omicron in South Africa was met with stiff resistance by health authorities, especially with the replicated version of Moderna as

> Further easing of restrictions came into effect on 23 March 2022, including dropping the requirement to wear masks outdoors though still required indoors in public vehicles and spaces, allowing proof of vaccination or a COVID-19 test not older than 72 hours as an alternative for entering certain venues, and reducing distancing to 1 metre except in schools. . . . Deaths were more decoupled from cases, likely due to high levels of population immunity from infection and/or vaccination. Eminent risk declined by mid-June 2022, and on 22 June 2022 all remaining health regulations regarding COVID-19 were ended.
> (Puren, 2022, *National Institute for Communicable Diseases*)

The US Omicron offensive though emerged not in the Trump era was a message about the high-minded desire of a developing country's leadership (the South African paradigm) to be very quick in addressing a disease of invasive proportions. This US Omicron environment does not evidence the South African successful struggle as far as the Omicron rampage was concerned. The following disclosure manifests the US initial challenges with the strain:

> Schools going virtual, airlines canceling flights, pharmacies and testing centers closing temporarily, shelves emptying in grocery stores because of transportation delays, blood donations dropping to crisis levels for the first time ever and the country's hospitals are becoming stretched. This is the US in the grip of the Omicron variant.
> (Schreiber, 2022, *The Guardian*)

The challenges of the pandemic notwithstanding, the South African Covid-19 epoch can be remembered for the country's frank and sincere considerations about humanity, all expressed through constructive, practical, and value-sensitive processes that were put in place to halt the plundering of the society by an air-borne invader, very much at variance with the politics-burdened American disposition to the health nuisance and inconvenience. A picture of the constructiveness of the nation's offensive, a blitzkrieg of actions, against coronavirus is cut in the information provided here:

> Officials in the Department of Health in Free State Province in South Africa beam with pride when talking about their response to COVID-19. Leadership, innovation, and partnerships, they say, have been key

to effectively tackling the pandemic and placed the province among those with the highest vaccination coverage in the country. Initially, the response to COVID-19 was centralized at the provincial level. Districts would gather data on paper, send the numbers to provincial level where officials would analyse it and feedback to the districts, which would then respond to an outbreak accordingly. But the delays in this lengthy process meant that by the time action was taken on the ground, infections were already high and deaths rising. "We realized quickly that this was not going to be sustainable," says Priscilla Monyobo, World Health Organization (WHO) provincial focal person. Key pandemic response measures including coordination, epidemiological surveillance, contact tracing, outbreak investigation, data management and analysis, infection prevention and control, community engagement as well as vaccination, were localized to the district level in July 2020. The decentralized approach led to faster outbreak detection and better targeted response. Standardized case investigation procedures were developed for district teams, for example, the time to start investigation was cut to 24 hours down from 72 hours when it was managed at the provincial level. Cluster outbreaks were identified quickly, and districts had a better understanding of the contexts of some of the outbreak trends.

(*World Health Organization*, 2022)

Conclusion

The Covid-19 imbroglio of the American presidency of Donald Trump is primarily a lesson in not how to be unpresidential in dealing with the people, and the need to be self-effacing, unassuming, and down-to-earth in matters of public safety and environmental sanity. Of secondary importance in this exegesis are the relevance and implications of Trump's handling of the pandemic to the Nigerian and South African social situations. Towards this end, the conceptual paradigms of Achille Mbembe's necropolitics and literary structuralism are considered pertinent in giving thoughtful critical considerations to the chequered reaction of the erstwhile president of the USA to the desolation caused by Covid-19, vis-a-vis its implications for growth in ruminations about the Nigerian and South African social, nay, political, systems.

From Ferdinand de Saussure's binary postulate to Northrop Frye's narrative categories, all absorbed in deconstructive strategies, Trump's engagement with the medical emergency explains itself as a development through self-aggrandizement, lack of seriousness and foresight, sensitivity to status, and a general zeal to upturn well-intentioned conventional beliefs about how well to protect the world from the clutches of unexpected environmental and health hazards. Achille Mbembe's pondering on necropolitics, as it impacts the use of sovereignty by a sovereign of any sort, especially in a democracy, echoes the abysmal sensitivity to power consciousness as deployed by Donald

Trump in his presidential obligations respecting devitalizing the viral adversity. The Nigerian and South African connections simply highlight the vagaries and multiplex dimensions of Donald Trump's responses to thoughts about social empowerment, political consciousness, and giving breath to environmental health concerns in a developing country.

References

Akwueh, E. (2022). Cameroon's Dam Not Responsible for Floods. *Nigerian Government.* https://von.gov.ng/cameroons-dam-not-responsible-for-floods-says-nigerian-government/#:~:text=Nigerian%20government%20has%20confirmed%20that,in%20many%20parts%20of%20Nigeria. Accessed 15 October 2022.

Aljazeera. (2022). South Africa Ends COVID Restrictions as Fifth Wave Fades. www.aljazeera.com/news/2022/6/23/south-africa-repeals-covid-rules-as-fifth-wave-fades. Accessed 10 December.

Amorighoye, T.A. (2020). COVID-19 Has Exposed the Education Divide in Nigeria. This Is How We Can Close It. *Education, Skills, and Learning.* www.weforum.org/agenda/2020/06/education-nigeria-covid19-digital-divide/. Accessed 15 October 2022.

APO Group. (2020). COVID-19 and Rural SA: The Good, the Bad and the Ugly. https://guardian.ng/apo-press-releases/covid-19-and-rural-sa-the-good-the-bad-and-the-ugly/. Accessed 11 December 2022.

Bagherioromi, A. (2021). How Volunteers in South Africa Are Combating a Global Pandemic: Young Volunteers in South Africa are Helping the Elderly in Their Communities Register for COVID-19 Vaccines. www.generationunlimited.org/stories/how-volunteers-south-africa-are-combating-global-pandemic#:~:text=Young%20volunteers%20in%20South%20Africa,register%20for%20COVID%2D19%20vaccinesandtext=As%20a%20third%20wave%20of,population%20of%20six%20million%20people. Accessed 11 December 2022.

BBC News. (2020). Coronavirus: Trump Stands by China Lab Origin Theory for Virus. www.bbc.com/news/world-us-canada-52496098. Accessed 22 July 2022.

Beckley Lovelace, Jr., B. and Breuninger, K. (2020). Trump Says He Takes Hydroxychloroquine to Prevent Coronavirus Infection Even Though It's an Unproven Treatment. www.cnbc.com/2020/05/18/trump-says-he-takes-hydroxychloroquine-to-prevent-coronavirus-infection.html. Accessed 10 August 2022.

Blog Post. (2022). Timeline of Trump's Corona Virus Responses, 2 March 2022. https://doggett.house.gov/media/blog-post/timeline-trumps-coronavirus-responses. Accessed 19 March 2022.

Burns, K. (2020). Trump's Seven Worst Statements on the Coronavirus. www.vox.com/policy-and-politics/2020/3/13/21176535/trumps-worst-statements-coronavirus. Accessed 27 March 2022.

Campbell, J. (2018). Controversy Surrounds Release of Most Dapchi Girls in Nigeria. www.cfr.org/blog/controversy-surrounds-release-most-dapchi-girls-nigeria. Accessed 15 October 2022.

Culler, J. (2001). *The Pursuit of Signs.* London: Routledge.

Das, S.S. and Sahana, D. (2019). *Book Review: Necropolitics. Theory in Forms, by Achille Mbembe.* Duke University Press. https://journals.sagepub.com/doi/full/10.1177/00020397221087747. Accessed 2 May 2023.

Dawsey, J. (2021). Poor Handling of Virus Cost Trump His Reelection, Campaign Autopsy Finds. www.washingtonpost.com/politics/poor-handling-of-virus-cost-trump-his-reelection-campaign-autopsy-finds/2021/02/01/92d60002–650b-11eb-886d-5264d4ceb46d_story.html. Accessed 12 March 2022.

Eagleton, T. (2008). *Literary Theory: An Introduction*. Minneapolis: University of Minnesota.

Elflein, J. (2023). Total Number of Cases and Deaths from COVID-19 in the United States as of September 9, 2022. www.statista.com/statistics/1101932/coronavirus-covid19-cases-and-deaths-number-us-americans/. Accessed 10 August 2022.

Encyclopedia Britannica. Personalism. www.britannica.com/topic/personalism. Accessed 16 June 2022.

Foundation for Investigative Journalism. (2022). Flashback: How Shetima's complacence led to Abduction of 276 Chibok School Girls. https://fij.ng/article/flash-back-how-shettimas-complacence-led-to-abduction-of-276-chibok-schoolgirls/. Accessed 1 November 2022.

Frye, N. (1957). *Anatomy of Criticism: Four Essays*. Princeton, NJ: Princeton University Press.

GQ. (2017). Donald Trump's Life in Pictures. www.gq-magazine.co.uk/gallery/donald-trump-pictures. Accessed 20 September 2022.

Haberman, M. and Sanger, D.E. (2020). Trump Says Coronavirus Cure Cannot "Be Worse than the Problem Itself". www.nytimes.com/2020/03/23/us/politics/trump-coronavirus-restrictions.html. Accessed 23 June 2022.

Haruna, A. (2018). Lai Mohammed Lied, Nigerian Govt Paid "Large Ransom" to Free #DapchiGirls – UN Report. www.premiumtimesng.com/news/headlines/280418-lai-mohammed-lied-nigerian-govt-paid-large-ransom-to-free-dapchigirls-un.html. Accessed 24 October 2022.

Immelman, A. and Griebie, A.M. (2020). The Personality Profile and Leadership Style of U.S. President, Donald J. Trump in Office. *Paper Presented at the 43rd Annual Scientific Meeting of the International Society of Political Psychology*, Berlin, Germany, 14–16 July 2020.

Jones, S. (2020). To Trump, America is Just a Series of Corporate Fiefdoms. https://nymag.com/intelligencer/2020/03/thanks-to-trump-coronavirus-will-make-some-people-rich.html. Accessed 29 April 2023 and 2 May 2023.

Kim, L.S. (2020). Law in a Time of Emergency: States of Exception and the Temptations of 9/11. *Journal of Constitutional Law*, 6(5): 1001–1083.

KPFK Radio. (2017). UNE's David Livingstone Smith Discusses Trump's Political Rhetoric on "KPFK" Radio. www.une.edu/news/2017/unes-david-livingstone-smith-discusses-trumps-political-rhetoric-kpfk-radio. Accessed 2 May 2023.

Kutsch, T. (2014). Anger Swells Against Nigeria Government in Response to Girl Abductions. http://america.aljazeera.com/articles/2014/5/5/nigeria-protestsboko.html. Accessed 24 October 2022.

Laughland, O. (2020). Trump Tells US "Relax, We're Doing Great" as His Virus Expert Says Worst Is Yet to Come. www.theguardian.com/world/2020/mar/15/trump-coronavirus-relax-were-doing-great-expert-worst-to-come. Accessed 15 July 2022.

Lemke, T. (2011). *Biopolitics: An Advanced Introduction* (pp. 9–10). New York: NYU Press.

Levin, B. (2020). Of Course the Trump Administration Warned Its Rich Pals How Bad Covid-19 Was Going to Get Bad While Telling the Public Everything Was

Fine. www.vanityfair.com/news/2020/10/trump-administration-warned-its-rich-pals-about-covid-19. Accessed 1 October 2022.

Maggi, H. (2020). Trade Adviser Warned White House in January of Risks of a Pandemic. www.nytimes.com/2020/04/06/us/politics/navarro-warning-trump-corona virus.html. Accessed 2 August 2022.

Marcel, G. (2009). *Homo Viator: Introduction to the Metaphysic of Hope*. Killington Way: St. Augustine's Press.

Mbembe, J.A. and Meintjes, L. (2003). Necropolitics. *Public Culture*, 15(1, Winter): 11–40. Duke University Press.

McKenzie, D. (2021). Southern Africa Hoped It Was Through the Worst of Covid-19. Then the Delta Variant Arrived. https://edition.cnn.com/2021/07/09/africa/south ern-africa-covid-delta-intl-cmd/index.html.

McQue, K. (2017). Nigeria Rejected British Offer to Rescue Seized Chibok Schoolgirls. www. theguardian.com/world/2017/mar/04/nigeria-declined-uk-offer-to-rescue-chibok-girls#:~:text=%E2%80%9CWe%20offered%20to%20rescue%20them,but%20 the%20Nigerian%20government%20declined.%E2%80%9Dandtext=The%20 girls%20were%20then%20tracked,the%20girls%20are%20still%20missing. Accessed 5 November 2022.

Norris, C. (1991). *Deconstruction: Theory and Practice*. London: Routledge.

Omarjee, L. and Magubane, K. (2020). Ramaphosa Announces South Africa's Biggest Spending Plan Ever to Fight Coronavirus. www.news24.com/Fin24/ramaphosa-announces-r500bn-support-package-adjustment-budget-for-coronavirus-20200421.

Onyeji, E. (2020). COVID-19: Governor Yahaya Bello Makes "False" Claims About "Mass Testing" in Kogi. www.premiumtimesng.com/news/headlines/433689-covid-19-governor-yahaya-bello-makes-false-claims-about-mass-testing-in-kogi.html. Accessed 15 October 2022.

Puren, A. (2022). Advisory on Measures to Control Covid-19 Following Lifting of Covid-19 Regulations. www.nicd.ac.za/wp-content/uploads/2022/06/Advisory-on-measures-to-control-COVID-19-following-lifting-of-COVID-19-regulations-28062022.pdf. Accessed 30 April 2023.

Reyes, M.V. (2020). The Disproportional Impact of Covid-19 on African Americans. www.ncbi.nlm.nih.gov/pmc/articles/PMC7762908/. Accessed 30 April 2023.

Rostan, T. (2020). Trump on Allowing Grand Princess Cruise Passengers to Disembark: 'I'd Rather Have Them Stay on, Personally. www.marketwatch.com/story/trump-on-allowing-grand-princess-cruise-passengers-to-disembark-id-rather-have-them-stay-on-personally-2020–03–07. Accessed 15 March 2022.

Schreiber, M. (2022). "The Economy Cannot Stay Open": Omicron's Effects Ricochet Across US. www.theguardian.com/us-news/2022/jan/12/us-omicron-cases-effects-schools-supply-shortage-hospitals. Accessed 10 December 2022.

Schwartz, R. (2023). The "Never Trump" Movement Is Back for Now. www.roll ingstone.com/politics/political-commentary/never-trump-movement-chris-christie-1234711652/. Accessed 1 May 2023.

Soyinka, W. (2021). *Trumpism in academe*. Ibadan: Bookcraft Publishing Services India Private Limited.

VOA. (2020). Africa Spared Worst of COVID-19 Pandemic by Working Together. www.voahausa.com/a/africa-spared-worst-of-covid-19-pandemic-by-working-together/5666179.html. Accessed 11 December 2022.

Ward, M. (2020). 15 Times Trump Praised China as Coronavirus Was Spreading Across the Globe. www.politico.com/news/2020/04/15/trump-china-coronavirus-188736. Accessed 22 March 2022.

Wordnik, Anachrony. www.wordnik.com/words/anachrony. Accessed 20 July 2022.

World Health Organization. (2022). Decentralized Response Boosts Free State Province's COVID-19 Fight. https://www.afro.who.int/countries/south-africa/news/decentralized-response-boosts-free-state-provinces-covid-19-fight#:~:text=The%20decentralized%20approach%20led%20to,managed%20at%20the%20provincial%20level. Accessed 10 December 2022.

Wright, E. (1998). *Psychoanalytic Criticism: A Reappraisal*. New York: Routledge.

Yong, E. (2020). How the Pandemic Defeated America. www.theatlantic.com/magazine/archive/2020/09/coronavirus-american-failure/614191/. Accessed 20 July 2022.

Conclusion

Towards Postcolonial Approaches to Health in a Globalized World

Olukayode A. Faleye, Tanimola M. Akande, and Inocent Moyo

In the introduction, it was emphasized that the overarching objective of this book is to illuminate the dominant knowledge and approaches to public health in so-called postcolonial Africa. If this is the case and if it is accepted that the aim of public health is to "improve the health of the whole community with an emphasis on protection, prevention of disease, and promotion of well-being" (Binns and Low, 2015: 5), it becomes evident that public health in Africa is haunted by not only the ghost of coloniality but also necropolitics. Concerning public health and necropolitics in postcolonial Africa, there is the recognition that other sections of the population are condemned to death, because their right to life based on the provision of adequate public health is confiscated by skewed policies which favour the elites and responds to the imperatives of the powerful. On the matter of coloniality, it needs reiteration that postcoloniality refers to a "temporal aftermath" and a "critical aftermath" (McEwan, 2009: 17), in which the former relates to the period after the end of colonial rule and the latter points to systems that sustain colonialism long after the end of colonial rule (Ndlovu-Gatsheni, 2013; Çalışkan and Preston, 2017). This critical aftermath

> survived the end of direct colonialism . . . it continues to affect the lives of people, long after direct colonialism and administrative apartheid have been dethroned. What, therefore, needs to be understood is . . . the invisible vampirism of technologies of imperialism and colonial matrices of power that continue to exist in the minds, lives, languages, dreams, imaginations, and epistemologies of modern subjects in Africa and the entire global South.
>
> (Ndlovu-Gatsheni, 2013: 11)

This necessarily brings to the fore the question of a proposal of how postcolonial approaches to health in Africa in a globalized world can be formulated and effectively implemented; hence this chapter which concludes this book is a modest attempt in that direction.

Indeed, Covid-19 should have taught the world that issues of public health are a global issue because all countries are interdependent based on

DOI: 10.4324/9781003429135-17

globalization and, therefore, there ought to be honest and globally coordinated efforts and strategies which promote public health for all people. More than that, the Covid-19 pandemic should have also taught the world about the limitations of modern science or the failure of modern science to respond to public health crises of global proportions (Moyo and Ndlovu-Gatsheni, 2023). This failure of modern science suggests that there are other epistemologies and/or knowledge which can be mobilized at a global level to respond to issues of public health. This brings to the fore the role that knowledge from Africa and the Global South in general can play. Indeed Ndlovu-Gatsheni (2020: 366) observes that

> Africa in particular and the Global South in general have the richest histories and experiences of epidemics and pandemics. This moment of the COVID-19 pandemic raises questions about the geopolitics of knowledge (which historical archive do we run to, who should learn from whom, and which epistemology is privileged?

Ndlovu-Gatsheni (2020) answers this question by suggesting that the time has come for African people and those of the Global South to lead and teach the rest of the world. This is based on that a significant number of African countries such as Liberia for example have experience in dealing with and responding to health pandemics and public health challenges. Based on this, it is proposed that one of the postcolonial approaches which can mobilized in responding to public health is African Indigenous knowledge systems. African nation-states and their government must realize that they have a rich indigenous knowledge systems and experiences from which they can and must draw in responding to and providing public health (Ndlovu-Gatsheni, 2020; Macamo, 2020, Pailey, 2020).

Thus, in the provision of health, African nation-states and government must move beyond the institutions and infrastructure that were built by colonial powers. It should be remembered that when the Empire built health institutions in many African countries in the name of public health, the intention was not driven by the need to provide health for all, but a selected few. It is indeed disturbing that many so-called postcolonial African nation-states still rely on colonial institutions and infrastructure to provide public health to all people when such infrastructure and institutions were not meant to provide public health for people. It is therefore not surprising that public health continues to be a challenge, and this is why we make the call for African nation-states to move beyond the institutions and infrastructure of the erstwhile colonizers, by adding those which promote indigenous knowledge systems in the context of public health. This is where African knowledge and experience in dealing with health pandemics and issues of public health can be mobilized. If this is done, Africans can and should stop looking to the West for solutions to the health pandemic and public health challenges (Pailey, 2020).

More than that, African countries should look at alternative ways of extracting their resources and developing their own industries. This is an important point, because the fact that Africa is a site for the extraction of natural resources which are exported to developed countries in North America and Western Europe has attracted multinational companies (MNCs) or transnational companies (TNCs) which extract raw materials but at the same time destroy the environment, which has implications on public health. What is important to note is that in many African countries, there is weak or no monitoring of the activities of multinational companies (see, e.g., Carmody, 2011). When public health problems arise, multinational companies are no longer accountable, the profits of raw material extraction have not benefited the people, but what remains on the ground is a degraded environment, sick, dead or dying African people. The point being made here is that there is a need to understand that public health issues on a local level are mediated by asymmetrical power relations at a global level. These asymmetrical power relations can be contested from below when African nation-states and their governments develop strategies which stop being a site for resource extraction, plunder, environmental degradation, leading to diseases and death. When the government fails to do something about the activities of multinational companies, ordinary groups and civil society organization ought to mobilize and hold these multinational companies accountable.

An inspiring case is that of ordinary people and concerned stakeholders in the Niger Delta in Nigeria, which have contested the activities of Shell and attempted to make it accountable (see Yusuf and Omoteso, 2016). Although they have not always been successful due to a combination of national and international alliances which work against them,

> the cases constitute an interesting milestone in the efforts of victims in the region to secure a remedy against the oil giant outside Nigeria's shores; a sign of the expanding recourse to this strategy across the Niger Delta. Such efforts have attracted the interests of international bodies and environmental rights groups who have accorded the local stakeholders substantial moral and legal support necessary to draw the attention of the world to their plight. This, in turn, is beginning to hold the oppressive hands of TNCs and making them pay for their environmental atrocities, notwithstanding TNCs' drive to escape justice by exploiting "legal forms" – the letters of the law – rather than its spirit.
> (Yusuf and Omoteso, 2016: 1383)

Climate change has shown the indivisibility of global destiny and the tragedy of the capitalist uneven mode of production. Extractive violence, the vacuity of material production and gluttonous consumption have found expression in climate stress characterized by natural disasters, the destruction of infrastructures and food insecurity. A formidable adaptive response to climate change requires bringing all hands on deck through an open knowledge translation that embodies inter-cultural dialogue (Tchoukaleyska et al., 2021). Here, African Indigenous knowledge could complement science in actualizing knowledge translation as engendered by collaborations that prioritize Africa's local realities in an interconnected world. Saving the world from the emerging climate Armageddon requires a governance system that transcends state-centric globality to a bottom-up glocality. In times of public health emergencies in Africa, non-state actors, including local churches, have provided public goods. Hence, there is an urgent need for a bottom-up rather than a top-down model that recognizes locally generated knowledge and solutions.

On the global stage, despite the changing dynamics of global power politics marked by the rise of China as a world power, South-South cooperation appears to be entangled in new centres of capitalist accumulation in South-east Asia. This is illustrative of the global economic structure where Africa's Look East Policy seems to guarantee the continuous exploitation of the region's natural resources and its designation as a dumping ground for hazardous products. Unfortunately, Africa bears the brunt of reckless resource exploitation. This implies that more initiatives to reverse climate stress should focus on Africa. Moreover, Africa deserves repatriation for the enduring extractive violence in the form of deliberate direct foreign green investment in the continent. In reversing climate stress and its associated displacement of people and social conflicts in Africa, the active involvement of the local actors in policy formulation and implementation is vital. Addressing the climate change-public health nexus would imply bridging the gap between town and gown, policy and practice as well as the geopolitical divide of the emerging global order.

References

Binns, C. and Low, W.-Y. (2015). What Is Public Health? *Asia Pacific Journal of Public Health*, 27(1): 5–6.

Çalışkan, G. and Preston, K. (2017). Tropes of Fear and the Crisis of the West: Trumpism as a Discourse of Post-Territorial Coloniality. *Postcolonial Studies*, 20(2): 199–216.

Carmody, P. (2011). *The New Scramble for Africa*. Cambridge: Polity Press.

Macamo, E. (2020). The Normality of Risk: African and European Responses to COVID-19. www.coronatimes.net/normality-risk-africa-europeanresponses/. Accessed 10 January 2021.

McEwan, C. (2009). *Postcolonialism and Development*. London: Routledge.

Moyo, I. and Ndlovu-Gatsheni, S.J. (Eds.). (2023). *The COVID-19 Pandemic and the Politics of Life*. London: Routledge.

Ndlovu-Gatsheni, S.J. (2013). Why Decoloniality in the 21st Century? *The Thinker: For Thought Leaders*, 48: 10–16.

Ndlovu-Gatsheni, S.J. (2020). Geopolitics of Power and Knowledge in the COVID-19 Pandemic: Decolonial Reflections on a Global Crisis. *Journal of Developing Societies*, 36(4): 366–389.

Pailey, R.N. (2020). Africa Does Not Need Saving During This Pandemic. https://www.alja zeera.com/opions/2020/13/africa-does-not-need-saving-during-thispandemic/?gb=true. Accessed 10 January 2021.

Tchoukaleyska, R., Richards, G., Vasseur, L., Manuel, P., Breen, S.-P., Olson, K., et al. (2021). Special Issue Introduction: Climate Change Knowledge Translation. *Journal of Community Engagement and Scholarship*, 13(3): Article 2. https://digitalcommons.northgeorgia.edu/jces/vol13/iss3/2.

Yusuf, H.O. and Omoteso, K. (2016). Combating Environmental Irresponsibility of Transnational Corporations in Africa: An Empirical Analysis. *Local Environment*, 21(11): 1372–1386.

Bibliography

Abayomi, A., Balogun, M.R., Bankole, M., Banke-Thomas, A., Mutiu, B., Olawepo, J., Senjobi, M., Odukoya, O., Aladetuyi, L., Ejekam, C., Folarin, A., Emmanuel, M., Amodu, F., Ologun, A., Olusanya, A., Bakare, M., Alabi, A., Abdus-Salam, I., Erinosho, E., Bowale, A., Omilabu, S., Saka, B., Osibogun, A., Wright, O., Idris, J., and Ogunsola, F. (2021). From Ebola to COVID-19: Emergency Preparedness and Response Plans and Actions in Lagos, Nigeria. *Globalization and Health*, 17(79). https://doi.org/10.1186/s12992-021-00728-x.

Abdullahi, A.A. (2011). Trends and Challenges of Traditional Medicine in Africa. *African Journal of Traditional Complementary and Alternative Medicines*, 8: 115–123. Department of Sociology South Africa.

Abidoye, R.O., Madueke, L.A., and Abidoye, G.O. (2002). The Relationship Between Dietary Habits and Body-Mass Index Using the Federal Airport Authority of Nigeria as the Sample. *Nutrition and Health*, 16(3): 215–227.

Abouyoub, Y. (2012). The Forgotten Culprit: The Ecological Dimension of the Darfur Conflict. *Race, Gender and Class*, 19(1/2): 150–176.

Adebowale-Tambe, N. (2020). COVID-19: Catholic Church Donates 425 Health Facilities as Isolation Centres. *Premium Times*. www.premiumtimesng.com/news/top-news/392311-covid-19-catholic-church-donates-425-health-facilities-as-isolation-centres-official.html?tztc=1. Accessed 11 March 2023.

Ademakinwa, J.A. (2012). *History of the Christ Apostolic Church: The Faith of our Fathers*. Grand Prairie: International Missions.

Adinlewa, T. and Ayara, M.G. (2019). Influence of Sexually Explicit Advertisements on the Sexual Values of Undergraduates of University of Lagos, Nigeria. *Novena Journal of Communication*, 9: 58–69.

Africa Center for Disease Control. (2022). Lassa Fever. https://africacdc.org/disease/lassa-fever/#:~:text=The%20overall%20case%2Dfatality%20rate,disease%20is%20not%20uniformly%20performed.

Aïach, P., Carr-Hill, R., Curtis, S., and Illsley, R. (1987). *Les inégalités sociales de santé en France et en Grande-Bretagne*. Paris: INSERM.

Akande, O.W. and Akande, T.M. (2020). COVID-19 Pandemic: A Global Health Burden. *National Postgraduate Medical Journal of Nigeria*, 27(3): 147–155. www.npmj.org/temp/NigerPostgradMedJ273147-50714_140514.pdf.

Akindele, F. and Adegbite, W. (1999). *Sociology and Politics of English in Nigeria*. Ile Ife: Obafemi Awolowo University Press.

Akwueh, E. (2022). Cameroon's Dam Not Responsible for Floods. *Nigerian Government*. https://von.gov.ng/cameroons-dam-not-responsible-for-floods-says-nigerian-government/#:~:text=Nigerian%20government%20has%20confirmed%20that,in%20many%20parts%20of%20Nigeria. Accessed 15 October 2022.

Aljazeera. (2022). South Africa Ends COVID Restrictions as Fifth Wave Fades. www.aljazeera.com/news/2022/6/23/south-africa-repeals-covid-rules-as-fifth-wave-fades. Accessed 10 December.

Allen, H. and Katz, R. (2010). Demography and Public Health Emergency Preparedness: Making the Connection. *Population Research and Policy Review*, 29(4): 527–539.

Alokan, A.J. (2011). *Christ Apostolic Church @ 90*. Ile-Ife: Timade Venture.

Alokan, P.O., Alabi, A.O., and Babalola, S.F. (2011). Critical Analyses of Church Politics and Crises Within the Indigenous Christianity in Nigeria. *American Journal of Social and Management Sciences*, 2(4): 360–370.

Altins, T.R. (1975). *Sexuality in the Movies*. Bloomington: Indiana University Press.

Amanze, C.U. (2006). The Socio-economic Impact of AIDS Scourge in Developing Countries. In Daura, M.M. (Eds.) *Nigeria's Technical Aid Corps: Issues and Perspectives*. Ibadan: Dokun Publishing House.

Amorighoye, T.A. (2020). COVID-19 Has Exposed the Education Divide in Nigeria. This is How We Can Close It. *Education, Skills, and Learning*. www.weforum.org/agenda/2020/06/education-nigeria-covid19-digital-divide/. Accessed 15 October 2022.

Anaemene, B.U. (2016). Health Sector Reforms and Sustainable Development in Nigeria: A Historical Perspective. *Journal of Sustainable Development in Africa*, 18(4): 50–66.

Anaemene, B.U. and Aworawo, D. (2014). Indigenous Health Practices in Africa. In Osuntokun, J. (Ed.) *African Peoples, Cultures and Civilization* (pp. 77–85). Ede: Redeemer's University Press.

Anoba, I.B. (2019). Misery Index Ranks Nigeria and South-Africa as Africas Most Miserable Countries. https://www.africanliberty.org/2019/04/11/misery-index-ranks-nigeria-and-south-africa-as-africas-most-miserable-countries/.

APO Group. (2020). COVID-19 and Rural SA: The Good, the Bad and the Ugly. https://guardian.ng/apo-press-releases/covid-19-and-rural-sa-the-good-the-bad-and-the-ugly/. Accessed 11 December 2022.

Aregbeshola, B.S. (2021). Towards Health System Strengthening: A Review of the Nigerian Health System From 1960 to 2019. *SSRN*, 14 January 2021. https://ssrn.com/abstract=3766017; http://dx.doi.org/10.2139/ssrn.3766017. Accessed 17 June 2021.

Asekun-Olarinmoye, O.S., Asekun-Olarinmoye, E.O., Adebimpe, W.O., and Omisore, A.G. (2014). Effects of Mass Media and Internet on Sexual Behaviour of Undergraduates in Osogbo Metropolis, South Western Nigeria. *Adolescence Health Medicine Therapeutics*, 5: 15–23. http://dx.doi.org/10.2147/AHMT.S54339.

Asogun, D.A., Adomeh, D.I., Ehimuan, J., Odia, I., and Hass, M. (2012). Molecular Diagnostics for Lassa Fever at Irrua Specialist Teaching Hospital, Nigeria: Lessons Learnt from Two Years of Laboratory Operation. *PLoS Neglected Tropical Diseases*, 6(9): e1839. https://doi.org/10.1371/journal.pntd.0001839.

Asuzu, M.C. (2004). The Necessity of a Health Systems Reform in Nigeria. *Journal of Community Medicine and Primary Health Care*, 16(1): 1–3.

Ate, A.A. (2008). *Media and Society*. Lagos: National Open University of Nigeria.

Ate, A.A. (2020). Hunting the Beast of Pornography in Nigeria: Theoretical, Legal and Ethical Perspectives. *Confluence Law Journal*, 3: 350–377.

Ate, A.A. (n.d.). *Theories of Mass Communication*. Ikeji-Arakeji: Joseph Ayo Babalola University (JABU).

Ate, A.A. and Ikerodah, J.O. (2019). Mass Communication Students Perception of Fake News Phenomenon in Nigeria. *Journal of Media, Communication and Languages*, 6(1): 131–141.

Ateh, F. (2018). *Seat of Thorns*. Yaounde: Nyaa Publishers.

Awuzie, S. (2021). Grief, Resurrection and the Nigerian Civil War in Isidore Diala's the Lure of Ash. *Tydskrif vir Letterkunde*, 58(2). https://doi.org/10.17159/tlv58i2.6793.

Ayegboyin, D. and Ishola, A. (1997). *African Indigenous Churches: An Historical Perspective*. Lagos: Greater Heights Publications.

Ayeni, A.O. (2016). Increasing Population, Urbanization and Climatic Factors in Lagos State, Nigeria: The Nexus and Implications on Water Demand and Supply. *Journal of Global Initiatives: Policy, Pedagogy, Perspective*, 11(2). http://digitalcommons.kennesaw.edu/jgi/vol11/iss2/6. Accessed 22 June 2022.

Bagherioromi, A. (2021). How Volunteers in South Africa are Combating a Global Pandemic: Young Volunteers in South Africa are Helping the Elderly in Their Communities Register for COVID-19 Vaccines. www.generationunlimited.org/stories/how-volunteers-south-africa-are-combating-global-pandemic#:~:text=Young%20volunteers%20in%20South%20Africa,register%20for%20COVID%2D19%20vaccinesandtext=As%20a%20third%20wave%20of,population%20of%20six%20million%20people. Accessed 11 December 2022.

Ball, S. (1998). Big Policies/Small World: An Introduction to International Perspectives in Education Policy. *Comparative Education*, 34(2): 119–129.

Balogun, A.S. (2010). HIV/AIDS Epidemic in the History of Nigeria, 1986–2007. *Journal of the Historical Society of Nigeria*, 19, 166–176.

Basure, H.S. (2021). *In Search of a Cure: Experiences in Alternative Medicine in Masvingo Urban, Zimbabwe*. Pretoria: University of Pretoria.

BBC News. (2021). Coronavirus in Nigeria: Goment Guidelines for Workers, Office and Business to Check Second Wave of Coronavirus, 4 January 2021. Accessed 7 February 2021.

BBC News. (2022). Coronavirus: Trump Stands by China Lab Origin Theory for Virus. www.bbc.com/news/world-us-canada-52496098. Accessed 22 July 2022.

Becker, C., Diakhaté, M., and Fall, A. (2008). Répartition des ressources et équité dans l'accès à la santé: une reproduction des inégalités. In Daffé, G. and Diagne, A. (dir.) *Le Sénégal face aux défis de la pauvreté. Les oubliés de la croissance* (pp. 81–108). Paris: Karthala, CRES and CREPOS.

Beckley Lovelace, Jr., B. and Breuninger, K. (2020). Trump Says He Takes Hydroxychloroquine to Prevent Coronavirus Infection Even Though It's an Unproven Treatment. www.cnbc.com/2020/05/18/trump-says-he-takes-hydroxychloroquine-to-prevent-coronavirus-infection.html. Accessed 10 August 2022.

Beinart, W. (2000). African History and Environmental History. *African Affairs*, 99(395): 269–302.

Berker, M. (2020). Nigeria Hit by Second Wave of Covid-19. *Anadolu Agency*, 18 December 2020. Accessed 7 February 2021.

Berlant, L. (2007). Slow Death. *Critical Inquiry*, 33(4): 752–762.

Bigliardi, S. (2019). The Advocates of Pseudoscience Are Not Monsters – But Pseudoscience is. *Skeptical Inquirer*, 43(6): 58–60.

Binns, C. and Low, W.-Y. (2015). What is Public Health? *Asia Pacific Journal of Public Health*, 27(1): 5–6.

Blog Post. (2022). Timeline of Trump's Corona Virus Responses, 2 March 2022. https://doggett.house.gov/media/blog-post/timeline-trumps-coronavirus-responses. Accessed 19 March 2022.

Bluemenstock, J.E. (2016). Fighting Poverty with Data. *Science*, 353(6301): 753–754.

Boettke, P. and Powell, B. (2021). The Political Economy of the COVID-19 Pandemic. *Southern Economic Journal*, 87(4), 1090–1106.

Boseley, S. (2014). Nigeria's Ebola Crackdown is an Example to the World, 20 October. www.theguardian.com/world/2014/oct/20/nigeria-ebola-crackdown-example-to-world. Accessed 12 November 2021.

Brooks, C., Lewis, R.W.B., and Warren, R.P. (1974). From Freud and Literature. In *American Literature: The Makers and the Making (Book D): 1914 to the Present* (pp. 2804–2812). New York: Martins Press.

Burns, K. (2020). Trump's Seven Worst Statements on the Coronavirus. www.vox.com/policy-and-politics/2020/3/13/21176535/trumps-worst-statements-coronavirus. Accessed 27 March 2022.

Burrows, M. and Engelke, P. (2020). *What World Post-Covid-19? Three Scenarios.* Washington, DC: Atlantic Council.

Çalışkan, G. and Preston, K. (2017). Tropes of Fear and the Crisis of the West: Trumpism as a Discourse of Post-Territorial Coloniality. *Postcolonial Studies*, 20(2): 199–216.

Calvet, L. (1999). *Pour une écologie des langues du monde.* Paris: Plon.

Calzadilla, A., Zhu, T., Rehdanz, K., Tol, R.S., and Ringler, C. (2013). Economywide Impacts of Climate Change on Agriculture in Sub-Saharan Africa. *Ecological Economics*, 93: 150–165.

Campbell, J. (2018). Controversy Surrounds Release of Most Dapchi Girls in Nigeria. www.cfr.org/blog/controversy-surrounds-release-most-dapchi-girls-nigeria. Accessed 15 October 2022.

Campbell, T. and Sitze, A. (2013). *Biopolitics: A Reader.* Durham: Duke University Press.

Carmody, P. (2011). *The New Scramble for Africa.* Cambridge: Polity Press.

Carter-Pokras, O., Zambrana, R.E., Mora, S.E., and Aaby, K.A. (2007). Emergency Preparedness: Knowledge and Perceptions of Latin American Immigrants. *Journal of Health Care for the Poor and Underserved*, 18(2): 465–481.

Catholic Caritas Foundation of Nigeria. (2022). HIV/AIDS Programme. www.caritasnigeria.org/. Accessed 11 March 2023.

Catholic Relief Services Nigeria Website. (2023). CRS in Nigeria. www.crs.org/our-work-overseas/where-we-work/nigeria. Accessed 22 March 2023.

Centers for Disease Control and Prevention (CDC). (2004). Imported Lassa Fever. *Morbidity and Mortality Weekly Report*, 53(38): 894–897.

Chavhunduka, G.L. (1998). *The Professionalization of Traditional Medicine in Zimbabwe.* Harare: ZINATHA.

Chiffoleau, S. (dir.). (2005b). *Politiques de santé sous influence internationale: Afrique, Moyen Orient.* Paris: Maisonneuve et Larose.

Chinweizu, Jemie, O., and Madubuike, I. (1980). *Decolonization of African Literature.* Enugu: Fourth Dimension Publishing Co Ltd.

Ciotti, M., Ciccozzi, M., Terrinoni, A., Jiang, W.C., Wang, C.B., and Bernardini, S. (2020). The COVID-19 Pandemic. *Critical Reviews in Clinical Laboratory Sciences*, 57(6), 365–388.

Colding, J. and Barthel, S. (2019). Exploring the Social-Ecological Systems Discourse 20 Years Later. *Ecology and Society*, 24(1). https://doi.org/10.5751/ES-10598-240102.

Connolly, C., Keil, R., and Ali, S.H. (2021). Extended Urbanisation and the Spatialities of Infectious Disease: Demographic Change, Infrastructure and Governance. *Urban Studies*, 58(2), 245–263.

Coulibaly, T., Islam, M., and Managi, S. (2020). The Impacts of Climate Change and Natural Disasters on Agriculture in African Countries. *Economics of Disasters and Climate Change*, 4: 347–364.

Culler, J. (2001). *The Pursuit of Signs*. London: Routledge.

Daffé, Z.N., Guillaume, Y., and Ivers, L.C. (2021). Anti-Racism and Anti-Colonialism Praxis in Global Health – Reflection and Action for Practitioners in US Academic Medical Centers. *The American Journal of Tropical Medicine and Hygiene*, 105(3): 557.

Das, S.S. and Sahana, D. (2019). *Book Review: Necropolitics. Theory in Forms, by Achille Mbembe*. Duke University Press. https://journals.sagepub.com/doi/full/10.1177/00020397221087747. Accessed 2 May 2023.

Davis, D.K. and Robinson, J.P. (1989). Newsflow and Democratic Society. In Constock, G. (Ed.) *Public Communication and Behaviour* (Vol. 2). Orlando, FA: Academic Press.

Dawsey, J. (2021). Poor Handling of Virus Cost Trump His Reelection, Campaign Autopsy Finds. www.washingtonpost.com/politics/poor-handling-of-virus-cost-trump-his-reelection-campaign-autopsy-finds/2021/02/01/92d60002–650b-11eb-886d-5264d4ceb46d_story.html. Accessed 12 March 2022.

De Juan, A. (2015). Long-term Environmental Change and Geographical Patterns of Violence in Dafur, 2003–2005. *Political Geography*, 45: 22–33.

DeBoom, M.J. (2021). Climate Necropolitics: Ecological Civilization and the Distributive Geographies of Extractive Violence in the Anthropocene. *Annals of the American Association of Geographers*, 111(3): 900–912. https://doi.org/10.1080/24694452.2020.1843995.

Dennis, E.E. (1991). The Media are Quite Powerful. In Dennis, E.E. and Merrikl, J.C. (Eds.) *Media Debates: Issues in Mass Communication*. London: Longman Publishing Group.

DeVries, J. (1981). Measuring the Impact of Climate on History: The Search for Appropriate Methodologies. In Rotberg, R. and Rabb, T. (Eds.) *Climate and History: An Interdisciplinary History*. Princeton: Princeton University Press.

Diala, I. (1997). *The Lure of Ash*. Lagos: Nok Publishers International.

Dries, A. (1998). *The Missionary Movement in American Catholic History*. Maryknoll, NY: Orbis Books.

Dumoulin, J. and Kaddar, M. (1993). Le paiement des soins par les usagers dans les pays d'Afrique subsaharienne: rationalité économique et autres questions subséquentes. *Sciences Sociales et Santé*, 81–199.

Eagleton, T. (1996) *Literary Theory: An Introduction*. Hoboken, NJ: Wiley Blackwell.

Eagleton, T. (2008). *Literary Theory: An Introduction*. Minneapolis: University of Minnesota.

Easton, D. (1965). *A Framework for Political Analysis*. Englewood Cliffs, NJ: Prentice-Hall Inc.

Ebereonwu. (2004). *The Unpublishable Poems*. Ibadan: Kraft Books Limited.

Edelman, M. (1988). *Constructing the Political Spectacle*. Chicago: University of Chicago Press.

Efem, B. (2021). Minister of Health Admonishes Nigerians to Continue to adhere to Covid-19 Protocols and Health Advisories to Avoid Second Wave of Infections. *Federal Ministry of Health*. Accessed 7 February 2021.

Egbule, J. (2015). A Health Protection Essay on the Outbreak of EBOLA in Nigeria 2014. MSc thesis. Public Health Protection, Faculty of Health and Social Sciences, University of Bedfordshire.

Ekaney, J. (2007). *Verdict of the Gods*. Cameroon: Buma Kor Publishers Ltd.

Ekeopara, C. and Azubuike, U. (2017). The Contributions of African Traditional Medicine to Nigeria's Health Care Delivery System. *Journal of Humanities and Social Science*, 22(5): 32–43. www.iosrjournal.org. Accessed 24 December 2022.

Ekwensi, C. (1962). *Burning Grass*. London: Heinemann.

Ekwuazi, H. (2009). *The Monkey's Eyes*. Ibadan: Kraft Books Limited.

Elflein, J. (2023). Total Number of Cases and Deaths from COVID-19 in the United States as of September 9, 2022. www.statista.com/statistics/1101932/coronavirus-covid19-cases-and-deaths-number-us-americans/. Accessed 10 August 2022.

Encyclopedia Britannica. Personalism. www.britannica.com/topic/personalism. Accessed 16 June 2022.

Ernst, E. (2000). Prevalence of Use of Complementary/Alternative Medicine: A Systematic Review. *Bulletin of the World Health Organization*, 78(2): 258–266.

Ernst, E. and Fugh-Berman, A. (2002). Complementary and Alternative Medicine: What Is It All About? *Occupational and Environmental Medicine*, 59(2): 140–144. BMJ Publishing Group Ltd. https://doi.org/10.1136/oem.59.2.140.

European Commission. (2021). *Joint Report by the Commission and the Council on Social Inclusion*. https://data.consilium.europa.eu/doc/document/ST-7301-2021-INIT/en/pdf.

European Expert Group on Sexuality Education. (2015) Sexuality Education – What Is It? *Sexuality, Society and Learning*, 16(4): 427–431.

Faleye, O.A. (2017a). Environmental Change, Sanitation and Bubonic Plague in Lagos, 1924–31. *International Review of Environmental History*, 3(2): 89–103.

Faleye, O.A. (2017b). Sociospatial Networks and Trans-Border Epidemic Surveillance in West Africa: The Ebola Outbreak of 2014–2015 in Perspective. *The Nigerian Health Journal*, 17(3): 61–69.

Faleye, O.A. (2019). Border Securitisation and Politics of State Policy in Nigeria, 2014–2017. *Insight on Africa*, 11(1): 78–93.

Faleye, O.A. (2023). COVID-19 Pandemic, Geopolitics of Health and Security Entanglement in West Africa. In Moyo, I. and Ndlovu-Gatsheri, S.J. (Eds.) *COVID-19 Pandemic and the Politics of Life*. London: Routledge.

Faleye, O.A. and Akande, T.M. (2019). Beyond "White Medicine": Bubonic Plague and Health Interventions in Colonial Lagos. *Gesnerus: Swiss Journal of the History of Medicine and Sciences*, 76(1): 90–110.

Fanon, F. (1964). *Toward the African Revolution*. New York: Grove Press.

Fassin, D. (1996). *L'espace politique de la santé: Essai de généalogie*. Paris: PUF.

Fassin, D. (2000). *Les enjeux politiques de la santé*. Paris: Karthala.

Fatunmole, M. (2022). Key Issues in Nigeria's New National Health Insurance Authority Act. www.icirnigeria.org/key-issues-in-new-national-health-insurance-authority-act.html. Accessed 6 August 2022.

Faye, S.-L. (2008). Devenir mère au Sénégal: des expériences de maternité entre inégalités sociales et défaillances des services de soins. *cahiers santé*, 18(3).

Federal Government of Nigeria (FGN). (1970). *Second National Development Plan 1970–1974: Programme of Post-War Reconstruction and Development*. Lagos: Federal Government Press.

Federal Government of Nigeria (FGN). (1975). *Third National Development Plan, 1975–1980*. Lagos: Federal Government Press.

Federal Government of Nigeria (FGN). (2022). *The National Health Insurance Authority Act*. Abuja: Federal Government Press.

Fidel, M., Kliskey, A., Alessa, L., and Sutton, O.P. (2014). Walrus Harvest Locations Reflect Adaptation: A Contribution from a Community-Based Observing Network in the Bering Sea. *Polar Geography*, 37(1): 48–68. http://dx.doi.org/10.1080/1088937X.2013.879613.

Fidler, D.P. (1997). The Public's Health in the Global Era: Challenges, Responses, and Responsibilities. *Indiana Journal of Global Legal Studies*, 5(1): 11–51.

FMOH. (2004). *Health Sector Reform Programme: Thrusts with a Logical Framework and Plans of Action, 2004–2007*. Abuja: Federal Ministry of Health.

Fogel, R. (1991). The Conquest of High Mortality and Hunger in Europe and America: Timing and Mechanisms. In Higgonet, P., Landes, D., and Rosovsky, H. (Eds.) *Favourites of Fortune: Technology, Growth and Economic Development Since the Industrial Revolution* (pp. 33–71). Cambridge: Harvard University Press.

Ford, J.V., Vargas, E.C., Finotelli, Jr., I., Fortenberry, J.D., Kismödi, E., Philpott, A., Rubio-Aurioles, E., and Coleman, E. (2019). Why Pleasure Matters: Its Global Relevance for Sexual Health, Sexual Rights and Wellbeing. *International Journal of Sexual Health*, 31(3): 217–230. https://doi.org/10.1080/19317611.2019.1654587.

Foucault, M. (1976 [2003]). *Society Must Be Defended: Lectures at the College de France, 1975–1976*. London: Allen Lane.

Foucault, M. (1978). *The Will to Knowledge: The History of Sexuality* (Vol. 1). London: Penguin.

Foucault, M. (1982). The Subject and Power. *Critical Inquiry*, 8(4): 777–795.

Foundation for Investigative Journalism. (2022). Flashback: How Shetima's complacence led to Abduction of 276 Chibok School Girls. https://fij.ng/article/flashback-how-shettimas-complacence-led-to-abduction-of-276-chibok-schoolgirls/. Accessed 1 November 2022.

Freud, S. (1986). Creative Writers and Day-Dreaming. In Kaplan, C. (Ed.) *Criticism: The Major Statements* (pp. 419–428). New York: St. Martin's Press.

Friant, S., Ayambem, W.A., Alobi, A.O., Ifebueme, N.M., Otukpa, O.M., Ogar, D.A., Alawa, C.B., Goldberg, T.L., Jacka, J.K., and Rothman, J.M. (2020). Eating Bushmeat Improves Food Security in a Biodiversity and Infectious Disease "Hotspot". *EcoHealth*, 17(1): 125–138.

Frye, N. (1957). *Anatomy of Criticism: Four Essays*. Princeton, NJ: Princeton University Press.

Gabriel, J.M. (2017). David Easton's "Authoritative Value Allocation" – Activating the Definition's Potential. *SSRN*, 1 February 2017. https://ssrn.com/abstract=2909910 or http://dx.doi.org/10.2139/ssrn.2909910.

Garba, H.M. (2020). Covid-19 and the Challenge of False Information. *Post Covid-19 Survival (Virtual) Seminar ECWA Theological Seminary, Igbaja and CBC Africa, Zoom (An Online Platform)*, 22–24 September.

Glissant, E. (1997). *Poetics of Relation* (trans. Betsy Wing). Ann Arbor, MI: The University of Michigan Press.

Goldstein, G. (1990). Urbanization, Health and Well-Being: A Global Perspective. *Journal of the Royal Statistical Society*, 39(2): 121–133.

GQ. (2017). Donald Trump's Life in Pictures. www.gq-magazine.co.uk/gallery/donald-trump-pictures. Accessed 20 September 2022.

Griffin, E.M. (2000). *A First Look at Communication Theory*. Boston: McGraw Hill.

Griffin, E.M. (2012). *A First Look at Communication Theory* (8th Edition). New York: McGraw Hill.

Gross, M. (1978). *The Psychological Society*. New York: Random House.

Guber, E. and Grube, J.W (2000). Adolescent, Sexuality and the Media. *Western Journal of Medicine*, 172(3): 210–214. https://doi.org/10.1136/ewjm.172.3.210.

The Guardian. (2021). Nigeria Now in Fourth Wave of COVID-19 Says NCDC, 21 December. https://guardian.ng/news/nigeria-now-in-fourth-wave-of-covid-19-says-ncdc/. Accessed 23 August 2022.

Guy, D. (1985). Notes Towards a Theory of Pornography. *Sun Magazine*. https://www.thesunmagazine.org/issues/115/notes-toward-a-theory-of-pornography. Accessed 15 February 2023.

Guy Emerson, R. (2019). *Necropolitics: Living Death in Mexico* (pp. 2–3). Berlin: Springer.

Haberman, M. and Sanger, D.E. (2020). Trump Says Coronavirus Cure Cannot "Be Worse than the Problem Itself". www.nytimes.com/2020/03/23/us/politics/trump-coronavirus-restrictions.html. Accessed 23 June 2022.

Hall, L.A. (2020). The Sexual Body. In *Medicine in the Twentieth Century* (pp. 261–275). London: Taylor & Francis.

Hamil, J. (2014). Porn Brand Behind 21st Century Playboy's Plans. A Hardcare Future for Journalism. *Forbes*, 16 May. https://www.forbes.com/sites/jasperhamill/2014/05/16/porn-brand-behind-21st-century-playboy-plans-a-hardcore-future-for-journalism/?sh=29f75b4a5567. Accessed 15 February 2023.

Happi, A.N., Happi, C.T., and Schoepp, R.J. (2019). Lassa Fever Diagnostics: Past, Present, and Future. *Current Opinion in Virology*, 37: 132–138. https://doi.org/10.1016/j.coviro.2019.08.002.

Harms, R. (1988). *Games Against Nature: An Eco-Cultural History of the Nunu of Equatorial Africa*. Cambridge: Cambridge University Press.

Harrington, R., Anton, C., Dawson, T.P., de Bello, F., Feld, C.K., Haslett, J.R., Kluvánkova-Oravská, T., Kontogianni, A., Lavorel, S., Luck, G.W., Rounsevell, M.D.A., Samways, M.J., Settele, J., Skourtos, M., Spangenberg, J.H., Vandewalle, M., Zobel, M., and Harrison, P.A. (2010). Ecosystem Services and Biodiversity Conservation: Concepts and a Glossary. *Biodiversity and Conservation*, 19(10): 2773–2790. http://dx.doi.org/10.1007/s10531-010-9834-9.

Harris, P. (1989). *A Cognitive Psychology of Mass Communication*. Hilldale, NJ: Lawrence Erlbaum Associates.

Haruna, A. (2018). Lai Mohammed Lied, Nigerian Govt Paid "Large Ransom" to Free #DapchiGirls – UN Report. www.premiumtimesng.com/news/headlines/280418-lai-mohammed-lied-nigerian-govt-paid-large-ransom-to-free-dapchigirls-un.html. Accessed 24 October 2022.

Hastings, A. (1989). *African Catholicism: Essays in Discovery*. London: SCM Press.

Hedstrom, J. and Harlsson, J. (2017). Consumers' Attitudes Toward Sexual Appeal in Advertising. Degree Thesis, Department of Business Administration, Technology and Social Sciences. Lulea University of Technology, Sweden. https://www.diva-portal.org/smash/get/diva2:1114476/FULLTEXT01.pdf.

Hibou, B. (1998). Economie politique du discours de la Banque mondiale en Afrique sub-saharienne. Du catéchisme économique au fait (et méfait) missionnaire. *Les Etudes du CERI*, 39: 46.

Hope, K.P. (1999). Managing Rapid Urbanization in Africa: Some Aspects of Policy. *Journal of Third World Studies*, 16(2): 47–59.

Hornberger, J. (2019). Who is the Fake One Now? Questions of Quackery, Worldliness and Legitimacy. *Critical Public Health*, 29(4): 484–493.

Hours, B. (2001b). Pour une anthropologie de la santé en sociétés. In Hours, B. (dir.) *Systèmes et politiques de santé. De la santé publique à l'anthropologie* (pp. 5–21). Paris: Karthala.

Hours, B. (dir.). (2001c). *Systèmes et politiques de santé: de la santé publique à l'anthropologie*. Paris: Karthala.

Inegbenebor, U., Okosun, J., and Inegbenebor, J. (2009). Prevention of Lassa Fever in Nigeria. *Transactions of the Royal Society of Tropical Medicine and Hygiene*, 104: 51–54.

Immelman, A. and Griebie, A.M. (2020). The Personality Profile and Leadership Style of U.S. President, Donald J. Trump in Office. *Paper Presented at the 43rd Annual Scientific Meeting of the International Society of Political Psychology*, Berlin, Germany, 14–16 July 2020.

Jahanger, A., Usman, M., Murshed, M., Mahmood, H., and Balsalobre-Lorente, D. (2022). The Linkages between Natural Resources, Human Capital, Globalization, Economic Growth, Financial Development, and Ecological Footprint: The Moderating Role of Technological Innovations. *Resources Policy*, 76(102569). https://doi.org/10.1016/j.resourpol.2022.102569.

Jobert, B. (1985). L'État en action. L'apport des politiques publiques. *Revue française de science politique*, 35(4): 654–682.

Jobert, B. (1992). Représentations sociales, controverses et débats dans la conduite des politiques publiques. *Revue française de science politique*, 42(2): 219–234.

Jones, J.L. (2010). "Nothing is Straight in Zimbabwe": The Rise of the kukiya-kiya Economy 2000–2008. *Journal of Southern African Studies*, 36(2): 285–299.

Jones, S. (2020). To Trump, America is Just a Series of Corporate Fiefdoms. https://nymag.com/intelligencer/2020/03/thanks-to-trump-coronavirus-will-make-some-people-rich.html. Accessed 29 April 2023 and 2 May 2023.

Jung, C. (1971). On the Relation of Analytical Psychology to Poetry. In Campbell, J. (Ed.), *The Portable Jung* (pp. 301–322). New York: The Viking Press.

Kaddar, M., Stierle, F., Schmidt-Ehry, B., and Tchicaya, A. (2000). L'accès des indigents aux soins de santé en Afrique subsaharienne. *Revue Tiers-Monde* (tome 41), 164: 903–925.

Kant, I. (1996). *The Metaphysics of Morals*. Cambridge and New York: Cambridge University Press.

Kaplan, C. (1986). *Criticism: The Major Statements*. New York: St. Martin's Press.

Kim, L.S. (2020). Law in a Time of Emergency: States of Exception and the Temptations of 9/11. *Journal of Constitutional Law*, 6(5): 1001–1083.

Kjekshus, H. (1977). *Ecology Control and Economic Development in East African History*. London: Heinemann.

Kutsch, T. (2014). Anger Swells Against Nigeria Government in Response to Girl Abductions. http://america.aljazeera.com/articles/2014/5/5/nigeria-protestsboko.html. Accessed 24 October 2022.

Lagos State Government. (n.d.). About Lagos. https://hos.lagosstate.gov.ng/about-lagos/.

Lambiase, J. and Reichert, T. (2003). *Sex in Advertising*. Mahwah, NJ: Lawrence Erlbaum Associates.

Lang, T. (2001). Public Health and Colonialism: A New or Old Problem? *Journal of Epidemiology & Community Health*, 55(3): 162–163.

Laughland, O. (2020). Trump Tells US "Relax, We're Doing Great" as His Virus Expert Says Worst is Yet to Come. www.theguardian.com/world/2020/mar/15/trump-coronavirus-relax-were-doing-great-expert-worst-to-come. Accessed 15 July 2022.

Leftwich, A. (2008). *Developmental States, Effective States and Poverty Reduction: The Primacy of Politics*. Geneva: United Nations Research Institute for Social Development.

Lemke, T. (2011). *Biopolitics: An Advanced Introduction* (pp. 9–10). New York: NYU Press.

Levin, B. (2020). Of Course the Trump Administration Warned Its Rich Pals How Bad Covid-19 was Going to Get Bad While Telling the Public Everything was Fine. www.vanityfair.com/news/2020/10/trump-administration-warned-its-rich-pals-about-covid-19. Accessed 1 October 2022.

Library of Congress Country Studies and CIA World Factbook. (1991). Nigeria History of Modern Medical Services. https://photius.com/countries/nigeria/society/nigeria_society_history_of_modern_me~10005.html. Accessed 28 February 2023.

Liverpool, J. (2004). Western Medicine and Traditional Healers: Partners in the Fight Against HIV/AIDS. *Journal of the National Medical Association*, 96(6). Atlanta, Georgia.

Lowes, S.R. and Montero, E. (2021). The Legacy of Colonial Medicine in Central Africa. *American Economic Review*, 111(4): 1284–1314. https://doi.org/10.1257/aer.20180284.

Macamo, E. (2020). The Normality of Risk: African and European Responses to COVID-19. www.coronatimes.net/normality-risk-africa-europeanresponses/. Accessed 10 January 2021.

Magesa, L. (1997). *African Religion: The Moral Traditions of Abundant Life*. Nairobi: Paulines Publications Africa.

Maggi, H. (2020). Trade Adviser Warned White House in January of Risks of a Pandemic. www.nytimes.com/2020/04/06/us/politics/navarro-warning-trump-coronavirus.html. Accessed 2 August 2022.

Marais, K. (2019). Calls for Pleasure: How African Feminists are Challenging and Unsilencing Women's Sexualities. *Agenda*, 33(3): 87–95.

Mararike, M. (2019). *Zimbabwe Will Never be a Colony Again! Sanctions and Anti-Imperialist Struggles in Zimbabwe*. Bamenda: Langaa RPCIG.

Marcel, G. (2009). *Homo Viator: Introduction to the Metaphysic of Hope*. Killington Way: St. Augustine's Press.

Matunhu, V., Matunhu, J., and Kalunta-Crumpton, A. (2019). Obtrusive Forms of Violence Against Young Women in Zimbabwe. *Violence against Women of African Descent: Global Perspectives*, 51.

Mbembe, J.A. (2003). Necropolitics. *Public Culture*, 15(1): 11–40.

Mbembe, J.A. (2019). *Necropolitics*. Durham: Duke University Press.

McCann, J.C. (1999). Climate and Causation in African History. *The International Journal of African Historical Studies*, 32(2/3): 261–279.

McEwan, C. (2009). *Postcolonialism and Development*. London: Routledge.

Mckenzie, D. (2021). Southern Africa Hoped It Was Through the Worst of Covid-19. Then the Delta Variant Arrived. https://edition.cnn.com/2021/07/09/africa/southern-africa-covid-delta-intl-cmd/index.html.

McQuail, D. (2000). *Mass Communication* (4th Edition). London: Sage Publication.

McQue, K. (2017). Nigeria Rejected British Offer to Rescue Seized Chibok Schoolgirls. www.theguardian.com/world/2017/mar/04/nigeria-declined-uk-offer-to-rescue-chibok-girls#:~:text=%E2%80%9CWe%20offered%20to%20rescue%20them,but%20the%20Nigerian%20government%20declined.%E2%80%9Dandtext=The%20girls%20were%20then%20tracked,the%20girls%20are%20still%20missing. Accessed 5 November 2022.

Means, A.J. (2022). Foucault, Biopolitics, and the Critique of State Reason. *Educational Philosophy and Theory*, 54(12): 1968–1969. Taylor & Francis.

Medard, J.-F. (2001). Décentralisation du système de santé publique et ressources humaines au Cameroun. *Bulletin de l' APAD*, 21. https://doi.org/10.4000/apad.35.

Mola, I., Onibokun, A., and Oranusi, S. (2021). Prevalence of Multi-Drug Resistant Bacteria Associated with Foods and Drinks in Nigeria (2015–2020): A Systematic Review. *Italian Journal of Food Safety*, 10(4): 9417. https://doi.org/10.4081/ijfs.2021.9417.

Moyo, I. and Ndlovu-Gatsheni, S.J. (Eds.). (2023). *The COVID-19 Pandemic and the Politics of Life*. London: Routledge.

Muiu, M. (2002). Globalisation and Hegemony: Which Way Africa. *Journal of Policy Studies*, 8(1): 68–88.

Muller, P. (1996). Présentation, cinq défis pour l'analyse des politiques publiques. *Revue française de science politique*, 46(1): 96–133.

Mumo, P.M. (2009). The Psychological Aspects of African Healing. *Hekima: Journal of Humanities and Social Sciences*, 4(1): 62–69.

Mumo, P.M. (2012). Holistic Healing: An Analytical Review of Medicine-Men in African Societies. *A Journal of the Philosophical Association of Kenya, New Series*, 4(1): 111–122. Nairobi: University of Nairobi.

Murewanhema, G. and Dzinamarira, T. (2022). The COVID-19 Pandemic: Public Health Responses in Sub-Saharan Africa. *International Journal of Environmental Research and Public Health*, 19(8): 4448. MDPI.

Murphy, D.R. (1997). *Mass Communication and Human Interactions*. USA: Houston Mifflin Company.

Muwonwa, N. (2021). "Subverting Controls": Historicising the Multi-dimensions of Female Youth Sexuality in Post-colonial Zimbabwe. In *Fending for Ourselves: Youth in Zimbabwe, 1980–2020* (pp. 158–172). Harare: Weaver Press.

Ndlovu-Gatsheni, S.J. (2013). Why Decoloniality in the 21st Century? *The Thinker: For Thought Leaders*, 48: 10–16.

Ndlovu-Gatsheni, S.J. (2020). Geopolitics of Power and Knowledge in the COVID-19 Pandemic: Decolonial Reflections on a Global Crisis. *Journal of Developing Societies*, 36(4): 366–389.

Ngalamulume, K. (2006). Plague and Violence in Saint-Louis-du-Sénégal, 1917–1920. *Cahiers d'étudesafricaines*, 183. https://doi.org/10.4000/etudesafricaines.6027.

Ngetcham. (2022). *Pour une Critique Archeologique des Arts et des Lettres*. Tampere: Atramenta.

Norris, C. (1991). *Deconstruction: Theory and Practice*. London: Routledge.

Nwabuzor, E. and Mueller, M. (1985). *An Introduction to Political Science for African Students*. London: Macmillan.

Nworgu, K.O. (2020). Mass Media and Premarital Sexual Behaviour of the Adolescents in Imo State Nigeria. *Edições Anteriores*, 7(17): 1257–1270.

Obayelu, A.E., Okoruwa, V.O., and Oni, O.A. (2009). Analysis of Rural and Urban Households' Food Consumption Differential in the North-Central, Nigeria: A Microeconometric Approach. *Journal of Development and Agricultural Economics*, 1(2): 018–026.

Odunze, E., Mikecz, O., Pica-Ciamarra, U., and Boussini, H. (2018). The Africa Sustainable Livestock 2050 Initiative. The Monetary Impact of Zoonotic Diseases on Society in Nigeria: Evidence from Four Zoonoses. Food and Agriculture Organisation. https://www.fao.org/documents/card/en/c/CA2146EN/.

Ogunbekun, I., Ogunbekun, A., and Orobatan, N. (1999). Private Health Care in Nigeria: Walking the Tightrope. *Health Policy and Planning*, 14(2): 174–178.

Ojaide, T. (1990). *The Fate of Vultures and Other Poems*. Lagos: Malthouse Press Ltd.

Ojakorotu, V. and Kamidza, R. (2018). Look East Policy: The Case of Zimbabwe – China Political and Economic Relations since 2000. *India Quarterly*, 74(1): 17–41.

Okafor, A.C., Igwesi, S.N., David, E.J., Okolo, V.K., and Agu, K. (2016). Presence of Bacteria with Pathogenic Potential Among Already-Used Toothbrushes from University Students. *American Journal of Life Science Researches*, 4: 16–20.

Okigbo, C. (2008). *Labyrinths and Path of Thunder*. Lagos: Apex Books Limited.

Okigbo, P. (2008). Foreword. In *Labyrinths and Path of Thunder*. Lagos: Apex Books Limited.

Oladimeji, A.M., Gidado, S., Nguku, P., Nwangwu, I.G., Patil, N.D., Oladosu, F., and Poggensee, G. (2015). Ebola Virus Disease–Gaps in Knowledge and Practice Among Healthcare Workers in Lagos. *Tropical Medicine & International Health*, 20(9): 1162–1170.

Oladele T.T., Olakunde, B.O., Oladele, A.O., Ugbuoyi, S., and Yamey, G. (2020). The Impact of COVID 19 on HIV Financing in Nigeria: A Call for Proactive Measure. *BMJ Global Health*, 5(5): e002718. https://doi.org/10.1136/bmjgh-2020-002718.

Olaniyan, R., Faleye, O.A., and Moyo, I. (Eds.). (2021). *Transborder Pastoral Nomadism and Human Security in Africa: Focus on West Africa*. London: Routledge.

Olukoju, A. (2003). *Infrastructure Development and Urban Facilities in Lagos, 1861–2000*. Ibadan: IFRA.

Omarjee, L. and Magubane, K. (2020). "Ramaphosa Announces South Africa's Biggest Spending Plan Ever to Fight Coronavirus. www.news24.com/Fin24/ramaphosa-announces-r500bn-support-package-adjustment-budget-for-coronavirus-20200421.

Omoruan, A., Bamidele, A., and Philips, O. (2009). Social Health Insurance and Sustainable Health Care Reform in Nigeria. *Ethno-Med*, 3(2): 105–110.

Onyema, C. (2012). Ecotrauma, Dis-Locations, Dis-Eases and Global Parables in Chika Uniqwe's the Phoenix. *Ogele* (Special Edition), 2: 41–58.

Orgah, A.E. and Orgah, O.J. (2015). Herbal Medicine in Nigeria: A Practice at the Clinical Crossroad. *South American Journal of Clinical Research*, 2(2). Tianjin, China.

Osaghae, E.E. (2002). *Crippled Giant: Nigeria Since Independence*. Ibadan: John Archers Publishers Ltd.

Oyewole, O. E. and Atinmo, T. (2015). Nutrition Transition and Chronic Diseases in Nigeria. *Proceedings of the Nutrition Society*, 74(4), 460–465.

Packard, R.M. (2020). Post-Colonial Medicine. In *Medicine in the Twentieth Century* (pp. 97–112). London: Taylor & Francis.

Packard, R.M., Cooter, R., and Pickstone, J. (2003). Post-Colonial Medicine. In *Companion to Medicine in the Twentieth Century* (pp. 97–112). London: Routledge.

Pailey, R.N. (2020). Africa Does Not Need Saving During this Pandemic. https://www.aljazeera.com/opions/2020/13/africa-does-not-need-saving-during-thispandemic/?gb=true. Accessed 10 January 2021.

Palinkas, L.A. and Wong, M. (2020). Global Climate Change and Mental Health. *Current Opinion in Psychology*, 32: 12–16.

Paul, J. (1987). *Sollicitudo rei socialis* [Encyclical Letter], 30 December. www.vatican.va/holy_father/john_paul_ii/encyclicals/documents/hf_jp-ii_enc_30121987_sollicitudo-rei-socialis_en.html. Accessed 19 March 2023.

Plato. (1986). The Ion. In Kaplan, C. (Ed.) *Criticism: The Major Statements* (pp. 17–20). New York: St. Martin's Press.

Poloma, M. (1982). *The Charismatic Movement: Is there a New Pentecost?* Boston: G. K. Hall and Co.

Popoola, D. (1993). Nigeria: Consequences for Health. In Aderanti, A. (Ed.) *The Impact of Structural Adjustment in Africa: Implications for Education, Health and Employment* (pp. 92–97). London: Heinemann.

Porta, M. (Ed.). (2014). *A Dictionary of Epidemiology* (6th Edition). New York: Oxford University Press.

Puar, J.K. (2001). *Terrorist Assemblages: Homonationalism in Queer Times* (pp. 32–79). Durham: Duke University Press.

Punch. (2022). Viral Video: NYSC Reacts to Corpers' Erotic Dance at Orientation Camp, 16 March.

Puren, A. (2022). Advisory on Measures to Control Covid-19 Following Lifting of Covid-19 Regulations. www.nicd.ac.za/wp-content/uploads/2022/06/Advisory-on-measures-to-control-COVID-19-following-lifting-of-COVID-19-regulations-28062022.pdf. Accessed 30 April 2023.

Raineri, L. (2020). Sahel Climate Conflicts? When (Fighting) Climate Change Fuels Terrorism. *European Union Institute for Security Studies, Brief*, 20: 1–8. www.jstor.org/stable/resrep28786. Accessed 25 April 2023.

Rainhorn, J.-D. and Burnier, M.-J. (dir.). (2001). *La santé au risque du marché: incertitudes à l'aube du XXIe siècle*. Paris: PUF.

Ramos, J.G.P., Garriga-López, A., and Rodríguez-Díaz, C.E. (2022). How is Colonialism a Sociostructural Determinant of Health in Puerto Rico? *AMA Journal of Ethics*, 24(4): 305–312.

Reyes, M.V. (2020). The Disproportional Impact of Covid-19 on African Americans. www.ncbi.nlm.nih.gov/pmc/articles/PMC7762908/. Accessed 30 April 2023.

Ridde, V. and Girard, J.-E. (2004). Douzeans après l'initiative de Bamako: constats et implications politiques pour l'équité d'accès aux services de santé des indigents africains. *Santé publique*, 41: 37–51.

Rokhmah, D. and Khorion, P. (2015). The Role of Textual Behaviour in the Transmission of HIV/AIDS in Adolescent in Coastal Area. *Procedia Environmental Sciences*, 23: 99–104.

Rostan, T. (2020). Trump on Allowing Grand Princess Cruise Passengers to Disembark: 'I'd Rather Have Them Stay on, Personally. www.marketwatch.com/story/trump-on-allowing-grand-princess-cruise-passengers-to-disembark-id-rather-have-them-stay-on-personally-2020–03–07. Accessed 15 March 2022.

Sandblom, P. (1989). *Creativity and Disease: How Illness Affects Literature, Art and Music*. Philadelphia: GB Lippincott Company.

Schreiber, M. (2022). "The Economy Cannot Stay Open": Omicron's Effects Ricochet Across US. www.theguardian.com/us-news/2022/jan/12/us-omicron-cases-effects-schools-supply-shortage-hospitals. Accessed 10 December 2022.

Schwartz, R. (2023). The "Never Trump" Movement is Back for Now. www.rollingstone.com/politics/political-commentary/never-trump-movement-chris-christie-1234711652/. Accessed 1 May 2023.

Sen, A. (1981). *Poverty and Famines: An Essay on Entitlement and Deprivation*. Oxford: Oxford University Press.

Senanu, K.E. and Vincent, T. (1976). *A Selection of African Poetry*. London: Longman Group Limited.

Shenjere-Nyabezi, P. (2022). Ethnoarchaeology of Cattle in Zimbabwe and Surrounds. *Oxford Research Encyclopedia of Anthropology*. https://oxfordre.com/anthropology/browse;jsessionid=1C199DD142AAD3FB8D25860CDF001364?page=5&pageSize=20&sort=titlesort&subSite=anthropology.

Shuaib, F., Gunnala, R., Musa, E.O., Mahoney, F.J., Oguntimehin, O., Nguku, P.M., Nyanti, S.B., Knight, N., Gwarzo, N.S., Idigbe, O., Nasidi, A., and Vertefeuille, J.F. (2014). Ebola Virus Disease Outbreak – Nigeria. *MMWR Morbidity and Mortality Weekly Report*, 63(39): 867–872.

Siahpush, M. (1999). Why Do People Favour Alternative Medicine? *Australian and New Zealand Journal of Public Health*, 23(3): 266–271.

Sinnerbrink, R. (2005). From Machenschaft to Biopolitics: A Genealogical Critique of Biopower. *Critical Horizons*, 6(1): 239–265.

Smith, A. (1776). *An Inquiry into the Nature and Causes of the Wealth of Nations*. Indianapolis: Liberty Classics.

Soyinka, W. (2021). *Trumpism in academe*. Ibadan: Bookcraft Publishing Services India Private Limited.

Suzuki, M. and Yang, S. (2022). Political Economy of Vaccine Diplomacy: Explaining Varying Strategies of China, India, and Russia's COVID-19 Vaccine Diplomacy. *Review of International Political Economy*, 1–26.

Swanson, W.M. (1977). The Sanitation Syndrome: Bubonic Plague and Urban Native Policy in the Cape Colony, 1900–1909. *Journal of African History*, 18(3): 387–410.

Swantz, L. (1990). *The Medicine Man among the Zaramo of Dar es Salaam*. Turku: Mai Palmberg.

Synge, R. (1993). *Nigeria: The Way Forward*. London: Euromoney Books.

Szmigiera M., (2021). Most Miserable Countries in the World 2020. https://www.statista.com/statistics/227162/most-miserable-countries-in-the-world/.

Tchoukaleyska, R., Richards, G., Vasseur, L., Manuel, P., Breen, S.-P., Olson, K., Curtis, J.C.C., and Vodden, K. (2021). Special Issue Introduction: Climate Change Knowledge Translation. *Journal of Community Engagement and Scholarship*, 13(3): Article 2. https://digitalcommons.northgeorgia.edu/jces/vol13/iss3/2.

Thomas, C.R., Gordon, I.J., Wooldridge, S., and Marshall, P. (2012). Balancing the Tradeoffs between Ecological and Economic Risks for the Great Barrier

Reef: A Pragmatic Conceptual Framework. *Human and Ecological Risk Assessment*, 18(1): 69–91. http://dx.doi.org/10.1080/10807039.2012.631470.

Thompson, L. (2008). Black Death. In Ackermann, M.E., Upshur, J.-H.L., Schroeder, M.J., Whitters, M.F., and Terry, J.J. (Eds.) *Encyclopedia of World History*. New York: Infobase Publishing.

Townsend, P. (1979). *Poverty in the United Kingdom: A Survey of Household Resources and Standards of Living*. London: Penguin.

Transparency International. (2021). Corruption Perception Index 2020. www.transparency.org/en/cpi. Accessed 19 June 2021.

Trilling, L. (1974). From Freud and Literature. In Brooks, C., Lewis, R.W.B., and Warren, R.P. (Eds.), *American Literature: The Makers and the Making (Book D): 1914 to the Present* (pp. 2804–2812). New York: St. Martin's Press

Ugah, A. (1991). *Colours of the Rainbow*. Lagos: Kraft Books Limited.

UNAIDS. (2004). The Media & HIV/AIDS: Making the difference. https://data.unaids.org/publications/irc-pub06/jc1000-media_en.pdf.

UNAIDS. (2020). Global HIV & AIDS Statistics-Fact Sheet. https://www.unaids.org/en/resources/fact-sheet.

UNESCO. (2018). International Technical Guidance on Sexuality Education. https://www.unfpa.org/sites/default/files/pub-pdf/ITGSE.pdf.

UNICEF. (2000). *The Progress of Nations*. New York: The United Nations Children's Fund (UNICEF).

UNICEF. (2021). Nigeria: Key Demographic Indicators. www.data.unicef.org/country/nga.

United Nations. (n.d.). What Is Climate Change. *Climate Action*. https://www.un.org/en/climatechange/what-is-climate-change. Accessed 24 April 2023.

United Nations. (n.d.). Poverty Eradication. https://www.un.org/development/desa/social perspectiveondevelopment/issues/poverty-eradication.html#:~:text=Poverty%20entails%20more%20than%20the,of%20participation%20in%20decision%2Dmaking.

Vanguard. (2014). Again, Tiwa, Patoranking Thrill Audience with Sensual Dance, 15 December.

Vanguard. (2020). Lassa Fever: What Makes Lagos a Bad Case, 22 February. www.vanguardngr.com/2020/02/lassa-fever-what-makes-lagos-a-bad-case/. Accessed 24 June 2021.

Villella, P.B. (2022). Disputing Epidemics, Public Health, and Alternative Therapies in Latin American History. *Latin American Research Review*, 57(1): 213–225.

VOA. (2020). Africa Spared Worst of COVID-19 Pandemic by Working Together. www.voahausa.com/a/africa-spared-worst-of-covid-19-pandemic-by-working-together/5666179.html. Accessed 11 December 2022.

Wade, A. (2006). Speech to the Nation, 3 April.

Walker, D.H., Mccormick, J.B., Johnson, K.M., Webb, P.A., Komba-Kono, G., Elliott, L.H., and Gardner, J.J. (1982). Pathologic and Virologic Study of Fatal Lassa Fever in Man. *American Journal of Pathologists*, 107: 349–356.

Ward, L.M., Erickson, S.E., Lippman, J.R., and Giaccardi, S. (2016). Sexual Media Content and Effects. *Oxford Research Encyclopedias*. https://oxfordre.com/communication/display/10.1093/acrefore/9780190228613.001.0001/acrefore-9780190228613-e-2;jsessionid=0478B1E29A79302E17CC69D7A286FDD4?rskey=75ihDR&result=9.

Ward, M. (2020). 15 Times Trump Praised China as Coronavirus Was Spreading Across the Globe. www.politico.com/news/2020/04/15/trump-china-coronavirus-188736. Accessed 22 March 2022.

Whiting, M. (2020). Pandemics and the Church: What Does History Teach Us?. *Campus News*, Dallas Baptist University. https://www.dbu.edu/news/2020/03/pandemics-and-the-church-what-does-history-teach-us.html.

Wimmer, R.D. and Dominick, J.R. (2000). *Mass Media Research: An Introduction.* London: Walsworth Publishing Company.

Winslow. (1920). *Primary Health System in Nigeria.* Lagos, Nigeria: Elmore Publishers.

Wogu, J.O., Chukwu, C.O., Nwafor, K.A., et al. (2019). Mass Media Reportage of Lassa Fever in Nigeria: A Viewpoint. *Journal of International Medical Research*, 48: 1–7.

Wordnik. Anachrony. www.wordnik.com/words/anachrony. Accessed 20 July 2022.

World Bank. (2023). GDP by Purchasing Power Parity: Sub-Saharan Africa, European Union, United States and China, 1990–2021 (Constant 2017 International $). *World Bank's World Development Indicators Database.* https://data.worldbank.org/indicator/NY.GDP.MKTP.CD? Accessed 26 April 2023.

World Bank. (n.d.). Climate Change by CO_2 Emissions (kt). https://data.worldbank.org/topic/climate-change?locations=ZG-EU-US-CN. Accessed 25 April 2023.

World Health Organization. (2014). Nigeria is Now Free of Ebola Virus Transmission. www.who.int/mediacentre/news/ebola/20-october-2014/en/index1.html. Accessed 11 March 2022.

World Health Organization. (2015). *Transforming Our World: The 2030 Agenda for Sustainable Development.* Geneva: World Health Organization. https://sustainabledevelopment.un.org/post2015/transformingourworld. Accessed 24 April 2023.

World Health Organization. (2022a). Decentralized Response Boosts Free State Province's COVID-19 Fight. www.afro.who.int/health-topics/coronavirus-covid-19/south-africa-bolsters-covid-19-response#carousel__slide4. Accessed 10 December 2022.

Worldometer. (2021). Coronavirus Updates. Accessed 16 December 2020 and 7 February 2021.

Wrathall, D.J., Bury, J., Carey, M., Mark, B., McKenzie, J., Young, K., Baraer, M., French, A., and Rampini, C. (2014). Migration amidst Climate Rigidity Traps: Resource Politics and Social-Ecological Possibilism in Honduras and Peru. *Annals of the Association of American Geographers*, 104(2): 292–304.

Wright, E. (1998). *Psychoanalytic Criticism: A Reappraisal.* New York: Routledge.

Yéléhé-Okouma, M., Pape, E., Humbertjean, L., Evrard, M., El Osta, R., Petitpain, N., Gillet, P., El Balkhi, S., and Scala-Bertola, J. (2021). Drug Adulteration of Sexual Enhancement Supplements: A Worldwide Insidious Public Health Threat. *Fundamental & Clinical Pharmacology*, 35(5): 792–807.

Yong, E. (2020). How the Pandemic Defeated America. www.theatlantic.com/magazine/archive/2020/09/coronavirus-american-failure/614191/. Accessed 20 July 2022.

Yusuf, H.O. and Omoteso, K. (2016). Combating Environmental Irresponsibility of Transnational Corporations in Africa: An Empirical Analysis. *Local Environment*, 21(11): 1372–1386.

Index